first place
4health

Bible Study Series

God's purpose
for you

Lucinda Secrest M

Published by Gospel Light
Ventura, California, U.S.A.
www.gospellight.com
Printed in the U.S.A.

Caution: The information contained in this book is intended to be solely for
informational and educational purposes. It is assumed that the First Place 4 Health
participant will consult a medical or health professional before beginning this or
any other weight-loss or physical fitness program.

Library of Congress Cataloging-in-Publication Data
First Place 4 Health Bible study series : God's purpose for you.
p. cm.
ISBN 978-0-8307-5212-6 (trade paper)
1. Spiritual life—Christianity—Textbooks. 2. Spirituality—Textbooks.
3. Weight loss—Religious aspects—Christianity—Textbooks.
I. Gospel Light Publications (Firm)
BV4501.3.F5693 2009
248.4—dc22
2009036917

Rights for publishing this book outside the U.S.A. or in non-English
languages are administered by Gospel Light Worldwide, an international
not-for-profit ministry. For additional information, please visit
www.glww.org, email info@glww.org, or write to Gospel Light Worldwide,
1957 Eastman Avenue, Ventura, CA 93003, U.S.A.

contents

foreword

There are many in-depth Bible studies on the market. The First Place 4 Health Bible studies are not designed for the purpose of in-depth study, but are designed to be used in conjunction with the rest of the program to bring balance into your life. Our desire is for each member to begin having a personal quiet time with God each day. This time alone with God should include a time of prayer, Bible reading and Bible study. Having a quiet time is a daily discipline that will bring the rich rewards of balance, which is something we all need.

God bless you as you begin this exciting journey toward a balanced life. God will richly bless your efforts to give Him first place in your life. Remember Matthew 6:33: "But seek first his kingdom and his righteousness, and all these things will be given to you as well."

Carole Lewis, First Place 4 Health National Director

---

about the author

Lucinda Secrest McDowell, a graduate of Gordon-Conwell Theological Seminary, is an international conference speaker and author of eight books, including *Role of a Lifetime, Spa for the Soul, Amazed by Grace* and *Quilts from Heaven*. She has also written for 50 magazines and been a contributing author to 25 other books. A wife and mother of four, Cindy writes and speaks from New England through her ministry, Encouraging Words that Transform. Cindy and her husband, Mike, have led a First Place 4 Health group at their church in Weathersford, Connecticut. She is also part of a First Place 4 Health group comprised of fellow authors and helps coordinate their annual gathering. Visit her website, **www.encouragingwords.net** or contact her at **cindy@encouragingwords.net**.

introduction

First Place 4 Health is a Christ-centered health program that emphasizes balance in the physical, mental, emotional and spiritual areas of life. The First Place 4 Health program is meant to be a daily process. As we learn to keep Christ first in our lives, we will find that He is the One who satisfies our hunger and our every need.

This Bible study is designed to be used in conjunction with the First Place 4 Health program but can be beneficial for anyone interested in obtaining a balanced lifestyle. The Bible study has been created in a five-day format, with the last two days reserved for reflection on the material studied. Keep in mind that the ultimate goal of studying the Bible is not only for knowledge but also for application and a changed life. Don't feel anxious if you can't seem to find the *correct* answer. Many times, the Word will speak differently to different people, depending on where they are in their walk with God and the season of life they are experiencing. Be prepared to discuss with your fellow First Place 4 Health members what you learned that week through your study.

There are some additional components included with this study that will be helpful as you pursue the goal of giving Christ first place in every area of your life:

- **Group Prayer Request Form:** This form is at the end of each week's study. You can use this to record any special requests that might be given in class.

- **Leader Discussion Guide:** This discussion guide is provided to help the First Place 4 Health leader guide a group through this Bible study. It includes ideas for facilitating a First Place 4 Health class discussion for each week of the Bible study.

- **Two Weeks of Menu Plans with Recipes:** There are 14 days of meals, and all are interchangeable. Each day totals 1,400 to 1,500 calories and includes snacks. Instructions are given for those who need more calories. An accompanying grocery list includes items needed for each week of meals.

- **First Place 4 Health Member Survey:** Fill this out and bring it to your first meeting. This information will help your leader know your interests and talents.

- **Personal Weight and Measurement Record:** Use this form to keep a record of your weight loss. Record any loss or gain on the chart after the weigh-in at each week's meeting.

- **Weekly Prayer Partner Forms:** Fill out this form before class and place it into a basket during the class meeting. After class, you will draw out a prayer request form, and this will be your prayer partner for the week. Try to call or email the person sometime before the next class meeting to encourage that person.

- **Live It Trackers:** Your Live It Tracker is to be completed at home and turned in to your leader at your weekly First Place 4 Health meeting. The Tracker is designed to help you practice mindfulness and stay accountable with regard to your eating and exercise habits. Step-by-step instructions for how to use the Live It Tracker are provided in the *Member's Guide*.

- **Let's Count Our Miles!** A worthy goal we encourage is for you to complete 100 miles of exercise during your 12 weeks in First Place 4 Health. There are many activities listed on pages 255-256 that count toward your goal of 100 miles. When you complete a mile of activity, mark off the box listed on the Hundred Mile Club chart located on the inside of the back cover.

- **Scripture Memory Cards:** These cards have been designed so you can use them while exercising. It is suggested that you punch a hole in the upper left corner and place the cards on a ring. You may want to take the cards in the car or to work so you can practice each week's Scripture memory verse throughout the day.

- **Scripture Memory CD:** All 10 Scripture memory verses have been put to music at an exercise tempo in the CD at the back of this study. Use this CD when exercising or even when you are just driving in your car. The words of Scripture are often easier to memorize when accompanied by music.

welcome to
God's purpose for you

At your first group meeting for this session of First Place 4 Health, you will meet your fellow members, get an overview of your materials and find out what you can expect at weekly meetings. The majority of your class time will be spent learning about the four-sided person concept, the Live It Food Plan, and how change begins from the inside out. You will also have a chance to ask any questions about how to get the most out of First Place 4 Health. If possible, complete the Member Survey on page 205 before your first group meeting. The information that you give will help your leader tailor the next 12 weeks to the needs of the whole group.

Each weekly meeting begins with a weigh-in for members. This will allow you to track your progress over the 12-week session. Your Week One weigh-in/measurement will establish a baseline of comparison so that you can set healthy goals for this session. If you are apprehensive about weighing in every week, talk with your group leader about your concerns. He or she will have some options for you to consider that will make the weigh-in activity encouraging rather than stressful.

The day after your first meeting, begin Week Two of this Bible study. This session, you and your group will learn how to know God's purpose for the physical, spiritual, mental and emotional aspects of your health so that you can achieve your goals and maintain them over the long haul. As you open yourself to the truth of Scripture and share your hopes and struggles with the members of your group during the next 12 weeks, you'll find yourself becoming the healthy child of God you are designed to be!

respond
wholeheartedly

SCRIPTURE MEMORY VERSE
Where there is no revelation, the people cast off restraint;
but blessed is he who keeps the law.
PROVERBS 29:18

Do you struggle with roller-coaster weight—reaching one goal only to slide back into old habits? Do you wonder if it's even possible to maintain a healthy life? Through the next weeks, as you work through *God's Purpose for You*, you will learn how to make positive changes based on God's power and plan—changes that will enable you to be transformed in each area of health: physical, spiritual, mental and emotional.

Some of us have already seen God work in and through us to bring about long-term weight loss and a healthier lifestyle. Even though we may have, at one time, "cast off restraint" out of defeat and discouragement, God brought us to the end of *our* way so that He could have *His* way in all four areas of our lives. As He gently (and sometimes not so gently) uncovered truths that needed to be addressed, we then began to embrace a balanced life.

Some of us have not yet experienced God at work in our lives, and long to learn how we can invite Him in. God created us inside and out and desires us to keep soul and body in balance. If one is ignored, the other part suffers. Whether you have already begun getting your life in balance or are just starting out, *God's Purpose for You* will be a guide to what God's Word has to say about the process.

Each of us is somewhere on the journey, echoing this phrase: "I'm not what I *wanna* be; I'm not what I'm *gonna* be . . . but praise God Almighty, I'm not what I *was!*" And praise Him, too, that we are not alone, but traveling together in a group. You may know the other members of your group well or you may be just getting acquainted. Whatever the case, remember that even though you come with differing agendas and backgrounds, you meet on equal ground at the foot of the cross. Jesus will meet each of you where you are and ask, "Do you want to get well?" Your response may just change your life forever.

The first step in any new endeavor is to take stock of where you are. The second step is to ask God to show you where He wants you to be, and how to get there. This is done through prayer and the study of God's Word. As you align your desires with His, committing to do what is necessary to achieve your goal, He promises to give you divine power to overcome any obstacles in your path. As you grow in strength and daily disciplines, you will be able to stand firm against the enemy of your soul, the one who is trying to keep you down and defeated, discouraged and depressed. Grasping tightly to God's truth and listening to His guiding voice, you can go forward with the assurance that your life doesn't have to be a roller coaster of highs and lows—you can live in balance and encourage others to do the same!

RUNNING WILD Day 1

Lord, give me a new vision of the balanced life You have for me, which will come as I follow Your will and Your way. As I embrace Your law, may I also rejoice in the blessing. In Christ's name, Amen.

Write out this week's memory verse from Proverbs 29:18.

_____

_____

_____

_____

_____

There are at least three major phrases in this week's memory verse, but the one that particularly stands out is "the people cast off restraint." The *New Living Translation* says it like this: "They run wild." Isn't that a statement of our time—people running wild, doing their own thing? Unfortunately, that lifestyle leads to excess, not balance. In Proverbs 29:18, what is the condition that sets us up to cast off restraint and run wild?

What do you think is meant by the word "revelation" here?

The Latin root of "revelation" is *revelare,* which means "to unveil." What valuable truth do you think God wants to unveil to you today so that you might live a more balanced life?

THE MESSAGE paraphrase of Proverbs 29:18 is, "If people can't see what God is doing, they stumble all over themselves." Can you relate to that? Some of us have a history of trying the "diet of the day," only to toss it aside the moment we trip up. No wonder nothing works. After so many stumbles, many of us just give up—or worse, we give in to whatever feels good. And, frankly, eating usually feels good. It's comforting. It numbs us to other things going on in our lives that we aren't ready to address or conquer. But ultimately, it leads to a cycle of shame, guilt and defeat.

Psalm 73 speaks to those of us caught in a vicious cycle of destruction. Like the psalmist, we can cry out to God for help. Turn to Psalm 73 and write verses 21-22 below.

_____

_____

_____

_____

_____

God gives four distinct promises to you in Psalm 73:23-24:

He promises to always be _____.

He promises to hold you _____.

He promises to guide you _____.

He promises to take you _____.

Proverbs 20:18 tells us to do something when we make plans. Why do you think this is important?

_____

_____

_____

_____

_____

As you read Psalm 73:23-26, write out phrases that you can remember to claim on your journey toward health and wholeness.

_____

_____

_____

_____

Father, thank You for never giving up on me, even when I have failed. Thank You for promises that remind me You are enough. Amen.

WHAT GOD REVEALS

Lord, open my eyes to see all that You have for me today. Help me understand that Your law is for my good. In Christ's name, Amen.

Yesterday we examined the consequences of having no clear vision of God's purpose and plan for us. This week's memory verse is quite clear that "without a vision, the people perish" (*KJV*). As a refresher, what sets people up to cast off restraint?

_____

_____

_____

_____

Is it possible that God has provided revelation, but that people aren't aware of it? Explain your answer.

_____

_____

_____

_____

_____

Sometimes we know what to do, we just choose not to do it. Other times we are truly ignorant and don't know the best path for our lives. The great news is that we never have to stay in the dark, whether by choice or because of ignorance, because God wants to show us His will and His way. The second half of this week's memory verse gives us a clue about how to seek God's revelation. How do you think keeping God's law can help us understand His revelation?

_____

_____

_____

_____

_____

Do you cringe when you read the phrase "God's law"? Often that phrase conjures up connotations of rigidity, but the truth is that following God's law, found in the Bible, is the way to live the abundant, amazing life we are created to live. These are not rules to keep us from having fun—they are the recipes for successful living. Why do you think we sometimes have a negative reaction to being "constrained," even when it's by God's laws?

_____

_____

_____

_____

The First Place 4 Health program offers guidelines for our benefit—suggestions for eating healthily, exercising regularly, committing Scripture to memory, studying the Bible, praying for others and sharing together. How do you feel about these guidelines? Is there one or more that is particularly difficult for you at this time?

_____

_____

_____

How do you think your success might be derailed or delayed if you decide not to follow that particular guideline?

_____

_____

_____

_____

God uses His Word to reveal His way for us. In Deuteronomy 10:12-13, we read what He asks of His people. List five things God reveals as His will for your life in those verses.

1. _____

2. _____

3. _____

4. _____

5. _____

Did you notice the last phrase? *All these requirements are for your own good.* Do you believe that? Why or why not?

_____

_____

_____

_____

Gracious God, You know I long to serve You with my whole heart. Help me make time to do all that is truly important today. In Christ's name, Amen.

Day
3

CHOOSING GOD'S WAY

Lord, I want to choose what's best, but often I fall back into unhealthy patterns. Please direct my paths today toward balance and blessing. In Christ's name, Amen.

Proverbs 29:18 says we are blessed when we keep the law. Keeping the law is a conscious choice. For instance, if God's law is found in God's Word, we can only know it if we study the Bible. For many centuries, Christ-followers have learned how to follow God's law by observing spiritual disciplines such as Bible study, devotional reading, prayer, Scripture meditation and memorization, worship and fellowship, journaling, communion and more. Such practices help us cultivate the habit of keeping God's law. And as we get in that habit, we become more like Jesus. This is called "sanctification."

Sanctification is a building process; it doesn't happen all at once. You chose to open your Bible study book today because you decided in your mind first (and the rest of you followed) to study God's Word and pursue balance in the four areas of health. You could have chosen otherwise. Congratulations!

Psalm 119 is the longest chapter in the Bible, and it's all about the benefits of choosing to keep God's law. Turn to verses 1-2 and explain how they echo this week's memory verse.

_____

_____

_____

_____

In what ways have you been blessed this week by practicing some of the spiritual disciplines mentioned above? Try to pinpoint at least one blessing in each of the four areas.

Physical	Mental
Spiritual	Emotional

Are there certain "triggers"—times of the day or places or even people—that make it difficult for you to choose to keep the law? If so, what are those triggers?

_____

_____

_____

_____

What does Psalm 119:30-32 say? Write these verses below.

_____

_____

_____

_____

Do any of the verbs in those verses, such as "chosen," "set my heart," "hold fast" and "run" describe your life in these early weeks of seeking a more balanced life? How?

_____

_____

_____

_____

If you read further in Psalm 119 to verses 33-39, the psalmist asks God to do eight things so that he might be blessed. List these below:

1. Teach me _____
2. Give me _____
3. Direct me _____
4. Turn my heart _____
5. Turn my eyes _____
6. Preserve my _____
7. Fulfill Your _____
8. Take away _____

Almighty God, You know what is best for my life and my health.
Thank You for guiding me through Your Word. In Christ's name, Amen.

Day 4 UNDERSTANDING AND OBEDIENCE

Lord, forgive me for the times I simply do not want to obey You
because following You means going against my own will. Please change
my attitude from rebellion to obedience. In Christ's name, Amen.

"Do you understand *why* I'm telling you not to jump on your bed?" Cindy asked her three-year-old daughter, after explaining that Maggie could get hurt.

"Yes, Mama," she meekly replied. But Maggie's understanding didn't lead to obedience; almost immediately, she jumped off the bed, landed on a bedpost and knocked out three bottom teeth. As they rushed to the pediatric orthodontist to have extensive work done, all Cindy could think was, *Maggie's disobedience sure is expensive!*

Sometimes we think that we understand why God has set forth certain guiding principles in His Word. But then our wills collide with His, and we begin to "negotiate"—to follow only the laws that seem appropriate or convenient to us at the time. Unfortunately, that lack of understanding, coupled with a lack of obedience, can cost us dearly.

God's law is for our best, just as the law prohibiting Maggie from jumping on the bed was for her best. But her will and her way won out; maybe because she thought her mother's restrictions were simply to prevent her from having fun, when they were actually to prevent her from hurting herself.

In what ways have you been like Maggie? Have you found yourself resisting something you knew God was asking you to do because it was too difficult or just not fun? What did you discover about doing things your way versus following God's way?

_____

_____

_____

_____

_____

Can you remember a time when your disobedience led to pain? If so, describe that situation below, noting the consequences of your actions.

_____

_____

_____

_____

_____

If you find yourself chafing against some of First Place 4 Health's guidelines, remember that those guidelines exist so that you might have a fuller and more balanced life—not so that you will be miserable! Choosing to follow these guidelines is your decision. In the space below, write the psalmist's decision stated in Psalm 119:59-60. Are you ready to make a similar commitment to the guidelines for a healthy life? Why or why not?

When you, like the psalmist, "consider [your] ways" (v. 59), what are the "ways" that got you where you are today?

The psalmist speaks of turning his steps to God's statutes (v. 59). To *repent* means to feel regret about past actions and change your ways or habits—literally, to turn from one thing and go in a totally different direction. From what do you need to turn your steps? How can choosing a different direction help you?

What will you immediately do today to obey God's law?

Lord, on this new day I am taking a determined step to follow You in complete obedience. Thank You for helping me change direction. Amen.

WHOLEHEARTED

Day
5

Lord, I desperately want my efforts to achieve long-lasting success. Please do whatever is necessary to help me persevere with power. Amen.

One of the reasons we often fail in pursuing weight management is that we "dabble" in the process, rather than going for it wholeheartedly. Yet committing completely is the only path to success, according to one woman. She recently discovered that following without reservations can be a lesson in humility.

In the past, Wanda used to pick and choose when it came to diet regimens. She'd say, "Well, I'm not following *XYZ* diet exactly; I've modified it to meet my own needs." But at her First Place 4 Health meeting, she felt the Lord prodding her with a Dr. Phil-like question: "How's that working for you?"

Her response is a testimony to growth: "Oops! After realizing that my 'modifications' were really just excuses, I committed to do everything the First Place 4 Health team recommended, just like a little child. As soon as I pried my fingers of control off the situation, it became a delight. And yes, I've memorized all four verses so far. It's coming to this as a child that's working for me."

There are many reasons to lose weight. Sometimes an event provides incentive, such as going to a class reunion or an upcoming family wedding. Other times, we are frightened by a medical diagnosis and we want to reverse the negative results of an unhealthy lifestyle. Occasionally, people at work or well-meaning friends and family members drop hints that crush our spirits and cause us to decide, I'll show them!

Although God uses varied ways to get our attention, reasons such as these don't usually get us very far. We begin halfheartedly and go down from there. To achieve anything truly important and long lasting, we must do it for the right reasons and with our whole hearts.

Read Psalm 119:10-11,145-149. What does the psalmist declare in verses 10-11? Write these verses below.

In these verses, what two things does the psalmist say about his heart in his endeavor to follow God's law?

Is there any part of your heart that is holding back from being fully committed to living differently based on God's will and God's way? If so, why?

Do you need God's help in committing wholeheartedly to Him? Write down verses 145-146 as a prayer to Him:

Gracious God, I am determined to be faithful for the long haul.
Help me to embrace You fully while I put Christ first in my life
and follow this new regimen. In Christ's name, Amen.

REFLECTION AND APPLICATION

*Lord, it's hard to face up to some of my behavior and beliefs from the past.
Help me recognize that You are with me in the hard times and that You will
accompany me on this journey. In Christ's name, Amen.*

Timmy was a precocious preschooler in the days before seatbelts and
child carseats. In fact, he loved nothing better than standing on the front
seat while his dad drove their big station wagon.

"Sit down, Timmy!" Dad would say.

"Don't wanna!" Timmy replied.

"I said *sit down*!" Dad emphasized, his voice rising with each word.

As little Timmy finally plopped down, he muttered stubbornly, "I may
be sitting down on the outside, but I'm still standing up on the inside!"

Timmy's actions were obedient, but his heart was not—his rebellious
spirit was saying, "You may get me to do this now, but when you're not
around, I will have my own way!"

In what ways might you have acted like Timmy with regard to God's
commands?

All this week, we have talked about wholeheartedly keeping God's law.
This week's memory verse, Proverbs 29:18, states, "Where there is no revelation, the people cast off restraint; but blessed is he who keeps the law."
In what ways has God blessed you by keeping His "law"—such as in the
area of maintaining a healthy lifestyle?

One definition of *surrender* is "giving up control," while another is "an act of willing submission to authority." Both of those definitions describe what God wants us to do with our body, heart, mind and spirit. What are some specific ways in which you have surrendered control of your life to God? Is there anything else He is calling you to surrender?

_____

_____

_____

_____

> *Thank You, heavenly Father, that Your mercies are new*
> *every morning. In Christ's name, Amen.*

Day 7 — REFLECTION AND APPLICATION

Lord, may my life reflect order and purpose and balance.
Thank You that I am discovering the tools to make that happen. Amen.

Did you learn something new about God's law this week? As you reflect on all you studied, complete this comparison chart as best you can:

Consequences of "running wild"	Benefits of living by God's law

In *God's Prayer Book,* Ben Patterson makes the following suggestion:

> Ask yourself, "How would I act if I believed there is treasure hidden in the Bible?" If you had in your hands a map showing where you could find great material treasure, wouldn't you apply yourself diligently to crack any code or language and overcome any mountain, weather, or foe to find the treasure? Ask the Lord to so fill you with the purity and sweetness of His law (like fine gold and honey) that your interior life will be transformed, that your every thought will reflect His character.[1]

Lucy decided to try an experiment: She would seek to satisfy her spiritual hunger before her physical hunger. Every morning, she woke up early and had a time of Bible study and prayer before breakfast. By noting in her journal one "sweet treat" from those sessions, she was able to make food and eating a secondary focus in starting her day. God's promises came first. After just one month, it became a habit!

"Taste and see that the LORD is good; blessed is the man who takes refuge in him" (Psalm 34:8). What "sweet treat" will you dine on from God's Word today? Read one of the following verses that contain a specific promise from God: Deuteronomy 31:8; Psalm 32:8; Matthew 11:28; 2 Thessalonians 3:3; James 1:5; 1 John 5:14-15. Now write below or in your journal what was "sweet" to you—God's gift to you today from His Word.

_____

_____

_____

_____

Almighty God, You satisfy me with good things. Thank You for all I'm learning from the Bible—may it satisfy my deep hunger. In Christ's name, Amen.

Note

1. Ben Patterson, *God's Prayer Book: The Power and Pleasure of Praying the Psalms* (Wheaton, IL: Tyndale House Publishers, 2008), p. 73.

Group Prayer Requests

4 first place
health

Today's Date: _____

Name	Request
Stacy	Joy D. her ears water behind her ears.
Mae	
Ann	
Susie	for her mom.
Joy	for Linda that God heals her

Results

_____
_____
_____
_____
_____
_____

desire
real change

SCRIPTURE MEMORY VERSE
*May he give you the desire of your heart
and make all your plans succeed.*
PSALM 20:4

What do you want? If you could reach deep into your soul and identify your greatest longing, what would it be? Now, be honest and give a true answer. Ask God to help you peel away the layers of your heart and show you what appears to be your most important desire, even if you don't totally understand the state of your heart right now.

My deepest desire is *to see my whole family saved, and healed + others also*

We live each day in response to our deepest desires. The good news is that, at least for the past two weeks, First Place 4 Health has been part of your life plan—and it's likely this choice reflects your deep desire to live a healthy life. You have invested time, energy and resources to draw closer to God and seek His way for your physical, mental, spiritual and emotional health. But now you may be at the point where the newness and excitement has faded and you need to commit to the journey of change. Do you really want change? As you look at your life (relationships, time with God, eating, exercise) do you see any areas that need revamping and retooling?

The next question is how much you want to change. Because unless you truly, deeply desire change with your whole heart, you will never be able to keep going through the confusing midst of it in order to emerge on the other side.

Change is hard. Even changes we choose can bring on almost insurmountable adjustments. But feelings of frustration and failure can and should lead us to the arms of Christ, who welcomes and comforts us with the knowledge that we don't have to live this new life alone. He is beside us each step of the way, guiding and empowering with divine provision!

Can you come before Him with a still and quiet spirit today, believing that God knows your desires and plans for necessary changes in the various areas of your life?

Day 1

WHAT IS YOUR DEEPEST DESIRE?

Lord, sometimes I don't even know what I should desire. Please help me to understand and pinpoint godly desires and dreams for my life. In Christ's name, Amen.

Some say that if you want to know what's truly important in a person's life, ask how that person spends his or her time and money. Your checkbook and your planner can be quite revealing. What do your checkbook and planner reveal about what's most important to you?

In the introduction to this week's study, what did you write as your deepest desire? If you don't know what it is, how will you know when God grants it?

Saving + healing my family and loved ones

Psalm 37:4-6 reminds us that even though there is often bad news all around, God will bring justice for His people in His own way and His own time. There is a caveat, however—something we need to do in order for that to happen. Read those verses and fill in the blanks, which are the actions we must take:

Delight _thyself_ _also in the Lord_
and he will give you the desires of your heart. _Commit thy way_
unto the Lord Trust also in him,
him and he will do this: He will make your righteousness shine like the dawn, the justice of your cause like the noonday sun.

What do you think is meant by "delight yourself in the Lord"?

Give him your whole life in prayer
And loving him first in all things
Commit your ways unto the Lord.
Trust him And it shall come to pass

What is one way you could do that today?

Trust in him to no him in personal
way.

Do you find that it is harder to "commit your way to the Lord" or to "trust Him"? Why?

no I think its the only way
we find peace within. I think I think
its easy, you have to be Commited

Heavenly Father, I do commit myself to You in a fresh way today. Please help me learn to trust You with every detail of my life. In Christ's name, Amen.

Day
2

DO YOU WANT TO GET WELL?

*Lord, I'm dizzy from living a roller-coaster lifestyle. You know my heart,
so please help me be willing to be willing. In Christ's name, Amen.*

God knows our hearts even when we're not sure what's happening deep down inside. Even now, He knows your hopes and dreams as you study *God's Purpose for You.* But while He recognizes that you are taking steps towards a more balanced life, you may still need to take stock of your full intentions and answer this question: "Do you want to get well?"

Read John 5:1-9. Many who visit Jerusalem today are surprised at the great depth of the pool called Bethesda, even though over the centuries, land has built up and there no longer remains a refreshing and healing spa as was present in Jesus' day. Who was gathered around the pool at Bethesda?

Impotent folk, Blind, halt, weathered,

One invalid had been there for a long time. How long had he waited for healing? Why had it been so long (see v. 7)?

*A Certain man was there, which
had an infirmity Thirty + eight years.
He was waiting for the water to
be troubled.*

This pool was believed to have healing powers whenever the waters were stirred up. However, unless someone carried this man and placed him in the stirred-up waters, he had no hope for healing. What do you think this man's state of mind was when Jesus approached him as he was lying helplessly by the pool?

hopless

Do you think Jesus knew why the man was there? Do you think Jesus knew what was in the man's heart? What did Jesus say to him (see v. 6)?

Jesus said unto him, Rise take up your bed & walk,

Sometimes we can get so used to being the way we are that it becomes part of our identity. We cling to what we know rather than taking the risk to pursue real change in our lives. In what ways might you be enslaved to the status quo and fearful of pursuing true change?

If Jesus were to ask you today, "Do you want to get well?" what would be your answer? Write down the words you would say to Him if you could.

Yes

How did the man respond (see v. 7)? Did he answer Jesus' question?

And immediately the man was made whole, And took up his bed, And walked

Jesus didn't argue with the man, but He did ask him to do something. What was that (see v. 8)?

take up your bed & walk

The first two words in verse 9 are: _And immediately_ Wow! What was the first thing the man did?

the man was made whole

Later, even though Jesus' healing on the Sabbath had been controversial, what did the man go on to do (see vv. 11 and 15)?

he that made me whole, the same said unto me, take up thy bed and walk

> *Dearest Jesus, I've been lying by the pool for so long and now I'm ready to answer You. Do whatever it takes—I want to get well! Amen.*

Day 3 — YOUR PLANS, GOD'S PLANS

Lord, too often I react rather than respond. My life in some areas is so haphazard that I'm spinning in circles. Please help me focus. Amen.

Are you a control freak? Do you love to write down plans and fill in your schedule for weeks, months and sometimes years in advance, secretly believing that if you write it down, somehow you can control it? Any of us who struggle with control issues should memorize the wisdom found in Proverbs 19:21. Write that verse below:

There are many devices in a man's heart, nevertheless, the counsel of the Lord that shall stand

God doesn't want us to offer Him our plans so that He can rubber stamp them with His approval and send us on our way. He does, however, want us to plan. And then He wants us to offer up those plans to Him as an act of relinquishment, believing in faith that He will either bless them or redirect us. What does this week's memory verse say about our plans? Why do you think we have a tendency to make so many of them?

When we put them in Gods hands, then we know his will And he sees by faith, thy secced

Why do you think First Place 4 Health includes the discipline of keeping a Live It Tracker?

to keep use Commeted to what we should be eating & What we shouldnt be excersig.

What have you observed about your eating plans as you've used your Live It Tracker?

you Can look back And see where You can do things better

A wise grandmother once remarked, "If you don't know where you're going, you'll get there every time!" How can using the Live It Tracker help you get where you want to go?

It keeps you on track,

Read Proverbs 16:9. Record what your role is and what God's role is:

In his heart _Devæseth his way;_

but the Lord _Directed his steps._

Can you think of a time when you made plans in your heart, plans you thought would be pleasing to God, only to have Him direct your steps in a totally different direction? What happened?

_____

_____

_____

_____

At some point in life, many of us encounter a season of unemployment. Perhaps you're one of those who are now in-between jobs. If you've been there or are there now, you know that the old saying is true: "God can't steer a parked car!" It's up to us to get it moving—filling out applications, interviewing, praying, networking and asking God to open doors or close doors as He directs. We have our part to do; just sitting around the house waiting for the right job to drop down from the sky isn't realistic. We can also apply this principle to our pursuit of balanced living. What do you see as your part for moving forward on your health journey?

doing something about it.

_____

_____

_____

What do you see as God's part?

Directing use in the right way.

_____

_____

As we grow closer to God through prayer, Bible Study, worship and obedience, the easier it will be to determine the purposes of His heart. Read Psalm 33:11. What does God promise in this verse?

the Counsel of the Lord standeth for ever, the thoughts of his heart to all generations,

As you begin to release your plans to God, you become a model of obedience to the next generation. If your child (or any young person) asked you today, "Does God really have a plan?" how would you respond?

yes he dose have a plan for our lifes

Lord, I am ready to give up control of my life. Fill me with the good things You have planned for me. Thank You for helping me move forward. Amen.

INNER TRANSFORMATION

Day 4

Lord, when I look in the mirror, I hardly recognize that person. Help me to get my outer body and inner soul aligned together in such a way that You may be glorified. In Christ's name, Amen.

At a First Place 4 Health Wellness Week in Texas, two women walked together each morning. They both walked slowly and stretched their limits as the week went on. The one from Kansas went back home and kept going and going and going, and when she showed up at Wellness Week the next year . . . there were 100 pounds less of her to walk each morning!

That was a huge accomplishment for only one year! But her outward transformation was really just a manifestation of the changes God had made in her inwardly. What a great perk! If we follow a lifestyle that puts Christ first, change will happen on the inside and outside.

Read Romans 12:1-2. Paul encourages us to offer ourselves to God in this passage. What words does he use to describe the offering of our bodies (see v. 1)?

Living *sacrifice holy acceptable unto God*
Holy and *acceptable unto God*
Your spiritual _____ _____ _____

Have you ever thought of your body in such a way? How does his description make you feel?

its a reasonable service unto God

In verse 2, Paul gives further instructions. What does he tell us we should and should not do? What will be the result of this choice?

be not conformed to this world
But be ye transformed by the
renewal of your mind

The word "transformed" in verse 2 comes from the Greek word *metamorphoo*, from which we also get our English word "metamorphosis." The transformation God desires is a process of morphing into Christlikeness, a total change from one thing to a distinct other. Where does this morphing start in us (see v. 2)?

that you may prove whats is
that good acceptable and perfect
unto God

We must first decide in our minds that we are ready, willing and able to meet the challenge. What if you magically lost all your excess pounds and were immediately outwardly transformed? Would your unchanged inner life have an effect on your ability to keep it off? How does your mind and heart need to change in order to be successful for the long haul?

_____

_____

_____

_____

Does Paul ask you to do anything in this passage that is too hard? Why?

_____

_____

_____

_____

Think about the areas in your mind and heart that need inner transformation. Offer these to God and ask Him to do the *metamorphoo* work in you—to change you from the inside out!

> *Heavenly Father, please help me get rid of those things in my mind and heart that hinder my spiritual growth. I lay my whole life before You and ask You to change me from the inside out. In Christ's name, Amen.*

EMPOWERED FOR SUCCESS
Day 5

> *Lord, without divine intervention, I'll never be successful in my efforts. Please grant me Your Holy Spirit power to persevere and prevail. Amen.*

At some point on your journey toward a balanced life, you may think, *This is just too hard. I can't do it. I just can't. I do well for a little while, then I give in to old patterns and feel like giving up all together. It's just too hard.* Hey, we've all been there, and many of us have given in to discouragement and despair at failing yet another attempt for lasting health. This usually happens because we're trusting in our strength alone.

Let's face it: some of us are pretty strong and can keep going for quite a while. But the truth is, lasting change is too difficult to accomplish in our own strength. That's why God sent the Holy Spirit—to empower every believer to accomplish far more than we ever could by ourselves.

Read Romans 15:13. What are two results of trusting in God?

_____

_____

_____

_____

Think about vacuuming. If you push and pull the vacuum back and forth across your carpet, it may leave trails through the fibers that make your floor appear clean. But if you don't plug your vacuum in, no dirt is removed! The same is true for your journey toward a whole and healthy life—you need power! Read 2 Corinthians 3:18. Here, Paul talks about us being transformed into Christ's likeness with an ever-increasing glory. From what source does transformation come to us, according to Paul?

_____

_____

_____

_____

Are you depending on God to change you through the power of the Holy Spirit, or have you been striving to do it on your own? What are three specific steps you can take to "plug in" today?

_____

_____

_____

_____

One of the most amazing truths about the life of faith is that God uses ordinary people to do extraordinary things. Take the apostle Paul, for example. Even though he had incredible intellectual credentials, they were not what he depended on to spread the Good News of Christ. Read 1 Corinthians 2:3-5. Why did he rely on the Spirit's power (see v. 5)?

_____

_____

_____

_____

Remember: you can be successful in your quest to know God's purpose, but it's up to you to decide to appropriate God's power and provision.

> *Lord, in every crisis of my life, You have been there for me. Thank You that, through Your power, I can now serve and succeed. In Christ's name, Amen.*

REFLECTION AND APPLICATION

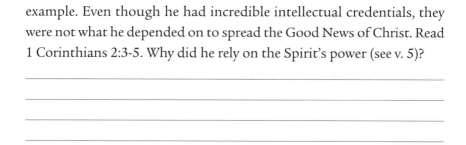

Day 6

> *Lord, I seek a fuller life than the one I'm currently living. Help me to cast aside anything that holds me back from Your best. In Christ's name, Amen.*

In *The Journey of Desire*, John Eldredge states that the reason most of us don't actually know what we want is that we're so unacquainted with our desire.[1] Is this true in your life? What is buried in your soul—buried because you dare not release it, just in case it's beyond reach and you're not sure you want to live with that kind of disappointment? Have you given up hope that your deepest desire might actually be from God, and therefore a gift? Are you willing to begin digging deep, chipping away at the protective walls that guard your heart from further disappointment and pain? What do you think you would uncover?

Is it possible that all too often we have sought *life* in all kinds of things other than God? Some of us, if we are brave enough to admit it, have even sought solace through eating—filling a void. When that happens, everything in us may be saying, *But I really want to eat that whole bag of potato chips—that seems like life to me right now.* God says, *I know you do, but it will kill you in the end. What you think is life is not. That's not the comfort [or love or significance] you are seeking. You'll wind up destroying yourself.* So, next time you find yourself seeking something other than God for spiritual satisfaction, remember to line up your desires with what God reveals to you in His Word.

What has God's Word—God's law—shown you is best for your life so far?

One definition of "desire" is *a longing for something.* "Longing" is a pretty strong word isn't it? It's more descriptive than just "wanting"—it connotes desperation for something. Do you long to be changed from the inside out? Share your feelings about this in a letter to God, your heavenly Father, either below or in your journal.

Jesus, help turn me from that which diminishes life to that which brings life. Give me hope that I can truly be changed. In Christ's name, Amen.

Day
7

REFLECTION AND APPLICATION

Lord, I want to believe that You have a plan and a purpose for my life. Help me to hold on to this promise. In Christ's name, Amen.

This week we learned that in order to embrace God's way, we must let go of seeking control. One practical exercise that may help you do this is to kneel by your bedside in prayer and open your hands. Envision yourself kneeling at the feet of Jesus as you release everyone and every situation to your Lord and Master, opening your hands to show that you're giving up control. (Of course, being in control is really an illusion—we never are in control; we just think we are.) With empty hands, you are ready to receive from Him exactly what He wants to give—His will, His way, in His time. It may help to repeat the words from the Lord's Prayer: "Your will be done. Your will be done."

This week's memory verse concludes with the phrase "and make all your plans succeed." What would that look like for you?

_____

_____

_____

_____

A promise from God is found in Jeremiah 29:11. What are the four purposes for you of God's plans, as outlined in this verse?

_____

_____

_____

_____

Spend some time today—at least 20 minutes—writing in your journal. Be specific about your goals (short term and long term) and your vision of your life when your desires have been fulfilled. As we progress together through *God's Purpose for You*, use your journal to write letters and prayers to God, and to record verses that become especially meaningful to you.

Gracious God, direct my thoughts and my pen as I seek to plan for success.
I will give my all and trust You with the results. In Christ's name, Amen.

Note
1. John Eldredge, *The Journey of Desire: Searching for the Life We've Only Dreamed Of* (Nashville, TN: Thomas Nelson Publishers, 2000).

Group Prayer Requests

4 first place
health

Today's Date: _____

Name	Request
Linda	sisters Grandson has a heart atack. Mattue
	Linda need prayer. for aleages. believe & have the faith.
Azuie	
	Be more loveing & careing
Joline	her daughter Surgery her moter + her dad in Hospise
Mae	
Jonie	wont make it till need help with her kids.
Susie	with my kids and Grandkids
Joy	her ears water behind her ears. Parkison test for agen orange Joy Franks. in alot of pain

Results

_____
_____
_____
_____
_____

love God totally

SCRIPTURE MEMORY VERSE
*Love the LORD your God with all your heart
and with all your soul and with all your strength.*
DEUTERONOMY 6:5

Are you a God-lover? Your first reaction to this question may be, "Of course I love God!" But, as this week's verse reminds us, our love for God should *consume* our whole being—heart, soul and strength.

Do you love God like that? The very first question in the Catechism, which some Christian traditions teach their children, is "what is the chief end of man?" The answer? "To glorify God and enjoy Him forever." What is God's ultimate purpose for us? To glorify Him in every area of our lives. But our purpose is also to enjoy God by loving Him totally.

In Deuteronomy 6:5, God commanded the Israelites to love Him with every part of them. What would loving God look like for you in these three areas?

All your heart: *with all thine heart*

All your soul: *And with Soul*
And with all my might

All your strength: *And My might*

Look up Mark 12:30. This verse is Jesus' answer to what question posed by what group of people (see vv. 28-29)?

scribs,
and thou shalt love the Lord thy God
with all thy heart. And with all thy
soul, And with all thy mint, And
with all thy strength; this is the first
this is the first commandment

Do you think what Jesus deemed as "the greatest commandment" might be important for you to obey too? If so, how do you think you are currently doing on "loving God totally"?

I defintly loving God totally, But
I still wante to love him even
more,

Day
1

WHAT GOD REQUIRES

Heavenly Father, help me today to love You with my heart,
soul and strength. In Christ's name, Amen.

Read Deuteronomy 10:11-13. Write out verses 12-13 below, underlining each word that indicates a command by God (there are five).

And now Isreal, what doth the Lord thy
God require of thee, But to fear the
Lord thy God, to walk in all his ways
And to love him, And to serve the Lord thy
God, with all thy heart and soul,
to keep the Commandments of the lord, And his
statutes, with I command. this day

In Deuteronomy 10, Moses is reminding the people of Israel how God gave him the Ten Commandments at Mount Sinai. Moses' job was to come back down from the mountain and do what (see v. 11)?

he stood before the people, that they may go in and possess the land

Then, in verses 12-13, Moses reminds the Israelites what they are required to do in order to inherit and inhabit the Promised Land. As you think of your health journey, what would you say is your "promised land"—the "place" you are seeking?

to fear him, to love him to walk in all his ways to love & serve him, with all my heart and soul,

How can you fulfill these commands and arrive in your promised land?

Fear the Lord: _thy God, to walk in all his ways_

Love Him: _And to serve the Lord_

Walk in His ways: _And to love him with all your heart & soul_

Serve the Lord with all your heart and soul: _____

_____

_____

_____

Observe the Lord's commands and decrees: _____

_____

_____

_____

Students of the Bible realize that when words and phrases are often re-peated, they indicate great importance. Throughout the Old Testament, God is adamant about His requirements for His people. Look up the fol-lowing verses and write below the commands in them.

Deuteronomy 11:1: _____

_____

_____

Deuteronomy 30:20: _____

_____

_____

Joshua 22:5: _____

_____

_____

Joshua 23:11: _____

_____

_____

Gracious God, thank You for going before me into the "promised land" of Your purpose in my life. May I follow with joy and obedience. Amen.

OBEDIENCE

Dearest Jesus, I want to obey You as an act of love. Help that love to flow from every part of me today. In Christ's name, Amen.

Read John 14:21. How does God know that we love Him?

_____

_____

_____

_____

_____

What does the disciple Jesus loved, John, say will happen to those who obey God's commands (see the second half of verse 21)?

_____

_____

_____

Having read some of God's commands yesterday, how would you evaluate your love of God, based on John's words?

_____

_____

_____

Why do you think it's so hard to love Him with every part instead of just those parts we are willing to surrender at any given time?

_____

_____

_____

Author Nancie Carmichael points out that "Jesus said we are to love Him with our body, mind, soul and spirit. That means loving Him with our whole selves, not just some splintered-off part."[1] One way to look at our response is to consider that we are like houses with four rooms—body, soul, mind and spirit—and to realize that to be a truly balanced person, we must tidy up each of these rooms every day. What will you do today in each of your four rooms to straighten them up?

Physical	Mental
Spiritual	Emotional

Thank You, Father, for helping me find balance in all areas of my life. In Christ's name, Amen.

Day 3 BELIEF SYSTEM

Almighty God, I know that Your commands are there for my good. May I follow them completely and joyfully. In Christ's name, Amen.

Read 1 John 5:1-3. In verse 1, John tells us another requirement for loving God: "believing that Jesus is the Christ." Describe when and where you first believed this.

_____

_____

_____

_____

John also adds a further proof of our love for God: those of us who love God will love others—by loving others, we will know we love God. How do you think loving others is an extension of loving God?

_____

_____

_____

_____

love God totally | 47

If you asked God to help you love others to demonstrate your love for Him, how do you think He might enable you to do this?

_____

_____

_____

_____

What does John remind us in verse 3?

_____

_____

_____

_____

Do you ever find God's commands to be a burden? If so, which ones?

_____

_____

_____

_____

What about the First Place 4 Health guidelines? Which ones seem burdensome to you and why?

_____

_____

_____

_____

It may be that your current belief system needs some overhauling so that you can come to believe what is true through God's Word. Carole Lewis, First Place 4 Health national director, shares that the secret for balanced health begins with the belief that *God is good*:

> God is good is one of the most far-reaching principles of the Bible, and it affects your life in ways that you may never have

imagined. . . . Nahum 1:7 says "The Lord is good, a refuge in times of trouble, He cares for those who trust in Him." That's the real answer to your goal of losing weight and becoming healthy. Start with the fact that God is good. He cares for you. The answer you're looking for encompasses not just taking off the pounds, but also living the life of purpose and hope you were meant to live. This is the life God calls you to live. And that life is well within your grasp.[2]

Do you truly believe, deep down, that God is good? If there is a part of you that is hesitant, why do you think you are reluctant to believe?

_____

_____

_____

_____

Gracious God, truly You are good and want good things for me.
Help me to believe that today and always. In Christ's name, Amen.

Day 4 · ACTIONS

Holy Spirit, reveal to me specific actions I can take today in order to show
my love as a follower of Jesus. In Christ's name, Amen.

Read 1 John 3:18-20. Verse 18 admonishes us to not love merely with _____ or _____ but with _____ and in _____.

The latest edition of *Merriam Webster's Collegiate Dictionary* includes a new word that comes to mind when I read this verse—frenemy. The definition of "frenemy" is "someone who acts like a friend but is really an enemy."[3] In other words, they may say all the right "friendly" words, but their "enemy" actions reveal otherwise.

In your journey toward balanced health, can you think of a time when you "talked the talk" but didn't "walk the walk"?

_____

_____

_____

_____

Mother Teresa, who ministered to the dying in Calcutta and organized the Missionaries of Charity in more than 52 countries, provided this insight into what it means to live by actions:

> I never look at the masses as my responsibility. I look at the individual. I can love only one person at a time. I can feed only one person at a time. Just one, one, one. As Jesus said, "Whatever you do to the least of my brethren, you do it to me." So I begin. I picked up one person. . . . The whole work is only a drop in the ocean. But if we don't put the drop in, the ocean would be one drop less. Same thing for you. Same thing in your family. Same thing in the church where you go. Just begin . . . one, one, one![4]

Read 1 John 3:19-20. How do these verses encourage you that loving God in both word and deed is possible, even if you have failed before?

_____

_____

_____

_____

Is your heart "at rest" in the presence of God? Take some time to sit in silence and just pour out your love to Him, not asking anything in return.

Heavenly Father, may I know that with every choice I make, I can make a difference in someone's life today. Let it be a good difference. Amen.

SOURCE OF LOVE

Lord, even though I've never actually seen You, I trust You for every need today and I want You to know that I love You. In Christ's name, Amen.

Read 1 John 4:7-16. What is the source of love, and to whom is it available (see vv. 7-8)?

_____

_____

_____

_____

In the first four days of this week, we have looked at the following areas. How are they spelled out again in this day's passage of Scripture?

Day 1—What God Requires (1 John 4:15-16)

_____

_____

_____

Day 2—Obedience (1 John 4:9)

_____

_____

_____

Day 3—Belief System (1 John 4:10,14)

_____

_____

_____

Day 4—Actions (1 John 4:11-12)

_____

_____

_____

If we don't love, what does this say about us and why (see v. 8)?

_____

_____

_____

What did God do to show how much He loves us (see vv. 9-10)?

_____

_____

_____

What should be our response to God's action of love (see v. 11)?

_____

_____

_____

Name two things that happen when we invite God's love into our hearts:

verse 12: _____

_____

_____

verse 15: _____

_____

_____

If you've experienced God's love in your life, when was the last time you shared that good news (see v. 14)? How will you testify to His love today?

_____

_____

_____

Gracious God, please clearly open a way for me to share Your love with someone today who desperately needs to know that good news. Amen.

REFLECTION AND APPLICATION

Lord, I am a fearful person much of the time and I don't understand why.
Will You deliver me from fear into faith? In Christ's name, Amen.

Read 1 John 4:17-21. What happens when God's love is made complete in us (see v. 17)?

_____

_____

_____

_____

Why do you think some people are afraid that God doesn't love them?

_____

_____

_____

What are your greatest fears today?

_____

_____

_____

_____

Why does fear have no place in the heart of anyone who loves God totally (see v. 18)?

_____

_____

_____

_____

How might being a fearful person affect your ability to be a loving person?

_____

_____

_____

Do you believe God is greater than your greatest fears? If you are afraid of anything in your First Place 4 Health journey, name those fears and pray right now that God will deliver you from them. Write your prayer below or in your journal.

_____

_____

_____

_____

In our goal to love God totally, we must also seek to be loving toward those around us. How is our love of God related to our love of others (see v. 20)?

_____

_____

_____

_____

One way of loving God is to love our brothers and sisters (see v. 21). Think of someone you have a hard time loving. Now, commit to pray for that person for each day this week and see if your heart toward them changes.

> *God, You know that sometimes loving others is hard for me. Help me today to love with the same love You have so graciously extended to me. Amen.*

REFLECTION AND APPLICATION

Day
7

> *Heavenly Father, sometimes I have a hard time understanding how You could love me unconditionally. Thank You for showing me every day that You really do! In Christ's name, Amen.*

First John 4:19 says, "We love because He first loved us." Do you know how much God loves you? As you familiarize yourself with the character of God, you will discover that His nature is Love—His love for us is a "sure thing"! Perhaps a study on the attributes of God will help you understand that God's love for you enables you to respond in kind with love for Him. God is with us along our journey toward balanced living and health. Like the old saying goes, "God loves us as we are, but loves us too much to let us stay there." Three words describe the greatness of who God is and what He can do. Look these up in a dictionary and write their definitions beside each characteristic of God.

Omniscient: _____

_____

Omnipotent: _____

_____

Omnipresent: _____

_____

Which one of these traits of God do you need to rely on or embrace in a special way this week?

_____

_____

_____

_____

As you continue to seek to love God totally, may these scriptural promises to you in the form of a love letter from God give you courage and strength to further embrace His purposes for your life:

Dear [your name],

Before the beginning of time, I knew you. I knew what color your eyes would be, and I could hear the sound of your laughter. Like a proud father who carries a picture of His daughter, I carried the image of you in My eyes, for you were created in My image. Before the beginning of time, I chose you. I spoke your name into the heavens and I smiled as its melody resounded off the walls of My heart.

You are Mine. My love for you extends farther than the stars in the sky and deeper than any ocean. You are My pearl of great price, the one for whom I gave everything. I cradle you in the palm of My hand. I love you even in the face of your failure. Nothing you can say or do can cause Me to stop loving you. I am ruthless in My pursuit of you. Run from Me—I will love you. Spurn Me—I will love you. Reject yourself—I will love you. You see, My love for you was slain before the foundations of the world and I have never regretted the sacrifice I made for you at Calvary.

When I see every part of who You are, I marvel at the work of My hands, for I whispered words of longing and desire and you came into existence. You are beautiful, and I take pleasure in you—heart, mind, and body. You are my desire. When you turn your head in shame and despise what I have made, still I reach for you with gentle passion. You are My beloved and I am yours.

Love, Your heavenly Father.[5]

Jesus, truly You are the Lover of my soul. I love you back,
now and forever. In Christ's name, Amen.

Notes

1. Nancy Carmichael, *Praying for Rain* (Nashville, TN: Thomas Nelson Publishers, 2001), p. 62.
2. Carole Lewis, *First Place 4 Health* (Ventura, CA: Gospel Light Publishers, 2008), pp. 25-26.
3. "frenemy," Merriam-Webster Online Dictionary, http://www.merriam-webster.com/dictionary/frenemy.
4. Mother Teresa, quoted in Susan Conroy, *Mother Teresa's Lessons of Love and Secrets of Sanctity* (Huntington, IN: Our Sunday Visitor Publishing Division, 2003), p. 205.
5. Regina Franklin, *Who Calls Me Beautiful?* (Grand Rapids, MI: Discovery House Publishers, 2004), pp. 44-45. (Based on Psalm 194:4; Song of Solomon 7:10,63; Isaiah 43:1; Matthew 13:46; Ephesians 1:4; 1 John 3:2; Revelation 13:8.)

Group Prayer Requests

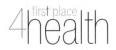

Today's Date: _____

Name	Request

Results

_____

_____

_____

_____

_____

_____

Week Five

stand strong

SCRIPTURE MEMORY VERSE
Put on the full armor of God so that you can take your stand against the devil's schemes.
EPHESIANS 6:11

For some, this week's memory verse may seem melodramatic—speaking of armor and the devil's schemes may feel, to some, like overreacting. For others, this verse is absolutely on target; they know that spiritual warfare is real in the life of anyone who truly wants to live for Christ. As you begin memorizing this verse and studying about God's purpose for us to stand strong, ask God to show you if the enemy of your soul (the devil) has established any strongholds in your life.

Beth Moore describes a stronghold as "anything that exalts itself in our minds 'pretending' to be bigger or more powerful than our God. It steals much of our focus and causes us to feel overpowered. Controlled. Mastered. Whether the stronghold is an addiction, unforgiveness toward a person who has hurt us, or despair over loss, it is something that consumes so much of our emotional and mental energy that abundant life is strangled—or callings remain largely unfulfilled and our believing lives are virtually ineffective."[1]

Strongholds are false, negative messages that hold us down and prevent us from conquering destructive patterns and lifestyles. Here are a few possible areas of strongholds. Prayerfully ask God to reveal to you if any of these (or others you could add in the blanks) are currently battling for your soul. Put a checkmark by any of the following strongholds at work in your life:

- ☐ Depression
- ☐ Anger
- ☐ Insecurity
- ☐ Unforgiveness
- ☐ Addictions
- ☐ Witchcraft
- ☐ Sexual impurity
- ☐ Fear

- ☐ Bitterness
- ☐ Jealousy
- ☐ Pride
- ☐ Shame
- ☐ Other: _____

_____

_____

_____

Day 1 PREPARED FOR BATTLE

Mighty God, please fight for me as I seek to demolish strongholds that have been in my life for a very long time. In Christ's name, Amen.

Are you finding it hard to keep the First Place 4 Health commitments to healthy eating, exercising, memorizing God's Word, praying for others and Bible study? Who do you think wants you to fail in each of these areas? Who do you think wants you to be victorious in each of these areas?

Read Ephesians 6:10-18. Who is our struggle against (see v. 12)?

_____

_____

_____

_____

God promises to fight life's battles for us and with us. He also gives us important tools for standing against all opposition. The apostle Paul loved God's people in the town of Ephesus, but he knew that they were sorely tempted to give in to the ways of the world and go against God's teachings. So Paul wrote to them using the imagery of battle and armor, hoping they would understand the concept of "putting on" spiritual armor each day as they sought to live for Christ. With that in mind, complete this table.

God's tool	Piece of Armor	What it does for us
Truth	Belt	
Righteousness	Breastplate	
Gospel of peace	Feet of readiness	
Faith	Shield	
Salvation	Helmet	
Word of God	Sword of the Spirit	

Verse 18 gives three final admonitions to remember as we go into battle. What are they?

1. _____

2. _____

3. _____

Several years ago, author John Eldredge was honored at a book convention with a large sword, as big as the one his *Braveheart* hero, William Wallace, used in Scotland many years ago. John loved it because it represented his core belief that all Christ-followers must be prepared to do battle for their very lives. "We are at war," he said:

This is a Love Story set in the midst of a life and death battle. Look around you at all the casualties strewn across the fields, the lost souls, the broken hearts, the captives. We must take this battle seriously—it is a war for the human heart. You have a crucial role to play. Many have underestimated their roles in the Story but that is dangerous. You will lose heart and you will miss your cues.[2]

Thank You, God, for all the armor You provide—I promise to put it on every single day! In Christ's name, Amen.

Day 2 — THE ENEMY

Dear Lord, speaking of Satan is sometimes frightening to me. Help me remember that You are more powerful. In Christ's name, Amen.

Read 1 Peter 5:8-11. In verse 8, Peter warns us to cultivate two important characteristics. What are they? Why are they important?

_____

_____

_____

_____

According to verse 9, what are we to do? Why?

_____

_____

_____

_____

Does verse 10 indicate that suffering might be a part of the Christian life? Why do you think this is (see Romans 8:17)?

_____

_____

_____

_____

What does verse 10 say that God will do for us in our suffering?

_____

_____

_____

_____

The book *Role of a Lifetime* reminds us that in every life story there is a villain who wants to win: "He wants to make your life so miserable, so full of fear, confusion, worry, and doubt that you will simply become paralyzed and unable to move forward in any kind of productive and redeeming way. If he can immobilize you, if he can demoralize you, if he can distract you from the role God has cast you in, he will have accomplished his purpose. . . . The one purpose of the enemy is the destruction of all God loves, particularly His beloved. That's you and me."[3] Who is the enemy of your soul and what has he done to you lately?

_____

_____

_____

_____

_____

Almighty God, the enemy may taunt and torture me, but by Your strength in my life, he will not win me over! In Christ's name, Amen.

GOD OFFERS STRENGTH

Day 3

Gracious God, today I feel weak, but I thank You that in my weakness, You are strong. In Christ's name, Amen.

Read Psalm 18:1-6. This psalm is a song of deliverance written by King David after the Lord rescued him from his enemies, which included the powerful King Saul (story found in 2 Samuel 22:1-51). According to Bible teacher Debbie Alsdorf, this psalm pictures God in five ways:

1. *God our rock.* He cannot be moved, even by our enemy. Solid and secure are we with God as our rock.
2. *God our fortress.* He is a place of safety.
3. *God our shield.* He is a barrier that comes between us and everything that passes through our life. Some describe this as having a "Father-filtered" life.
4. *God the horn or strength of our salvation.* Our salvation or deliverance doesn't rest on me. It rests on the strength of God; therefore, it is secure.
5. *God our stronghold.* If we need help or provision, we are to look to God. He is the One who holds us with strength that cannot be measured, for He alone is mighty and powerful above all else. We can trust in Him and in His strong grip on our lives.[4]

Which of these pictures of God do you need most on your journey toward health? Why?

_____

_____

_____

_____

Which of these pictures of God gives you most comfort and hope today, and why?

_____

_____

_____

_____

In *That Incredible Christian*, A. W. Tozer reminds us that God wants to give each of His children divine strength to stand against any enemy: "The purest saint at the moment of his greatest strength is as weak as he was before his concession. What has happened is that he has switched from his little human battery to the infinite power of God. He has quite literally exchanged weakness for strength, but the strength is not his, it flows into him from God as long as he abides in Christ."⁵ Have you taken hold of God's strength today? What can you do to plug into that power?

_____
_____
_____
_____

Thank You for being my Stronghold, my Rock and my Fortress today as I stand up against those who would discourage or distract me from knowing my true life's purpose. In Christ's name, Amen.

GOD LIFTS AND SUSTAINS
Day 4
Lord, when I am deep in the pit, please lift me up so that I may move forward with purpose and power. In Christ's name, Amen.

Read Psalm 18:16-19. List the verbs that describe what God did for King David:

verse 16: _____
verse 16: _____
verse 16: _____
verse 17: _____
verse 18: _____
verse 19: _____
verse 19: _____
verse 19: _____

Which of these actions do you need God to do in your life today, and why?

_____
_____
_____
_____

Read Psalm 18:30-36, in which David continues to praise God for making him strong. Write down phrases of praise:

verse 30: _____

verse 30: _____

verse 30: _____

verse 31: _____

verse 31: _____

verse 32: _____

verse 32: _____

verse 33: _____

verse 33: _____

verse 34: _____

verse 34: _____

verse 35: _____

verse 35: _____

verse 35: _____

verse 36: _____

verse 36: _____

Did you get all 16 on David's list? Wow! Now, write your own litany of praise to God, below or in your journal, for how He has helped you thus far in seeking to be healthy in all four areas of your life. For example, "You have helped me drive past fast-food takeout windows without ordering," or "You have wakened me early each morning so I could do my Bible study."

_____

_____

_____

_____

Gracious God, I am amazed and so thankful for new disciplines and activities in my life. Thank You for giving me power. In Christ's name, Amen.

GOD GIVES COURAGE

Day 5

Heavenly Father, may I always trust You to help me when I falter and fail. In Christ's name, Amen.

Read Joshua 1:6-9. Why do we need courage? Because fear is alive and well as we pursue balanced health. People fear what will happen if they don't lose the weight they need to lose, or they fear losing weight and then gaining it all back again. Mostly, people dread failure after so many attempts at change.

Do you sometimes struggle with fear? What are you most afraid of?

_____

_____

_____

_____

_____

Carole Lewis suggests that we need constant reminders to live in trust and dependence on God, believing that He will give us courage to fight fear and anxiety. She suggests:

1. Choose to obey God and leave the consequences of life to Him.
2. Recognize that God is greater than your circumstances.
3. Ask God to make you aware of His presence.
4. Praise God for delivering you from your fears.[6]

For each of these four steps, write down a specific action you can take to follow through on fighting fear:

Choose to obey God and leave the consequences of life to Him.

_____

_____

_____

Recognize that God is greater than your circumstances.

_____

_____

_____

Ask God to make you aware of His presence.

_____

_____

_____

Praise God for delivering you from your fears.

_____

_____

_____

Carole also notes that as you apply these four steps to your life and hold them in your heart, you will find yourself more able to conquer the obstacles of fear in your life, whether it concerns weight loss or anything else.

Father, thank You for always standing beside me through whatever comes my way. In Christ's name, Amen.

Day
6

REFLECTION AND APPLICATION

Great are You, Lord, and Your strength makes me strong. Hallelujah! In Christ's name, Amen.

Read Philippians 4:12-13. "Strong woman." "Strong man." Do you identify with that description? Why or why not?

_____

_____

_____

_____

Strength is more than firm bodies and toned muscles (although that's important too, and hopefully you're building those). According to Paul, the "secret of being content in every situation" is what (see v. 13)?

_____

_____

_____

_____

In what areas are you most discontented?

_____

_____

_____

_____

Does focusing on those areas make you stronger or weaker? Why?

_____

_____

_____

_____

A. W. Tozer once observed, "It is often said that we become like the person we spend the most time with. In fact, we do pick up their mannerisms and values as a part of our relationship with them. The same is true of our relationship with God. The more we spend time with Him the more we become like Him. Perhaps He is leading us to lay aside less important things that take up our time so we could and would spend that time with Him."[7] What do you think God may be calling you to lay aside in order to get to know Him better?

_____

_____

_____

_____

Today, take time with the God of all strength. Soak up His presence. Bask in His love. And echo Paul's words in verse 13: "I can do everything through him who gives me strength."

Heavenly Father, may nothing in this world come before my devotion to and delight in You. In Christ's name, Amen.

Day 7

REFLECTION AND APPLICATION

Master, help me to draw close to You each day so that I will always be prepared for unexpected battles. In Christ's name, Amen.

Since we're studying battle imagery all week, it might be instructive to look at some of the greatest warriors of all time—those from the Roman Empire. The shields of Roman soldiers were 4 feet by $2^1/_2$ feet, rectangular, and made of several layers of coated wood. Fiery darts would go into the shields and be put out. Helmets were of bronze; they were very heavy but extremely protective. It is said that during the heyday of the Roman Empire, the soldiers carried out daily maneuvers even in peace time, giving their all so that they would be prepared physically and mentally to withstand battle when it came.

The historian Josephus said, "No confusion breaks their customary formation, no panic paralyzes, no fatigue exhausts them. By their military exercises, the Romans instill into their soldiers fortitude not only of body, but also of soul."[8] Unfortunately, most historians agree that Rome eventually brought about its own downfall. Edward Gibbon reports that during the reign of Emperor Gratian, these rigorous disciplines were relaxed. Soldiers said the armor was too heavy, so they didn't use their shields and helmets. And because they didn't practice for battle each day, when the fighting actually came, they were weak and unprepared.[9]

In your battle of life, do you sometimes find the armor burdensome? Does the shield of faith sometimes feel too heavy? Are you tempted to compromise your faith at your workplace, with your social circle, or online? Has your sword dulled from disuse? Are you staying in the Word of God and learning it in your heart so that you can know what God wants and how to live?

As Beth Moore writes, "God has handed us two sticks of dynamite with which to demolish our strongholds: His Word and prayer. What is more powerful than two sticks of dynamite placed in separate locations? Two strapped together. Prayer keeps us in constant communion with God, which is the goal of our entire believing lives."[10] As Christ-followers, we have been equipped with what we need to prevail. No matter what we do, we must remember to hold on to prayer and Bible study as powerful instruments for standing strong!

Spend some time today praying God's Word, "strapping together" the two sticks of powerful dynamite God has provided you. A great place to start is the Psalms, many of which are prayers or testimonies about God's power and care. Find a psalm that speaks into your mind and heart today, and write it in your journal. When you feel attacked or under siege in the next week, use your dynamite! Pray that psalm and stand strong.

Almighty God, I pray today believing You can do what You say,
and that is the greatest power in the world. In Christ's name, Amen.

Notes

1. Beth Moore, *Praying God's Word* (Nashville, TN: B&H Publishers, 2000), p. 3.
2. John Eldredge, *Epic* (Nashville, TN: Thomas Nelson Publishers, 2004), p. 100.
3. Lucinda Secrest McDowell, *Role of a Lifetime: Your Part in God's Story* (Nashville, TN: B&H Publishers, 2008), p. 73.
4. Debbie Alsdorf, *Restoring Love* (Colorado Springs CO: David C. Cook Publishers, 2001), p. 25.
5. A.W. Tozer, *That Incredible Christian* (Camp Hill, PA: Christian Publications, 1986), p. 33.
6. Carole Lewis, *The Divine Diet* (Ventura, CA: Gospel Light Publishers, 2004), p. 195.
7. A.W. Tozer, *Gems from Tozer* (Camp Hill, PA: Christian Publications, Inc., 1979).
8. Flavius Josephus, *The Jewish War*, vol. III (Harvard University Press, 1997), p. 27.
9. Edward Gibbon, *History of the Decline and Fall of the Roman Empire*, vol. III (New York, Harper & Brothers Publishers, 1880), p. 238.
10. Moore, *Praying God's Word*, p. 6.

Group Prayer Requests

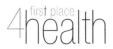

Today's Date: _____

Name	Request

Results

_____

_____

_____

_____

_____

_____

receive
divine power

Scripture Memory Verse
*His divine power has given us everything we need
for life and godliness through our knowledge of him
who called us by his own glory and goodness.*
2 Peter 1:3

"You've got what it takes!" is a popular slogan these days. The very phrase seems empowering and energizing. Do you ever wonder if you have "what it takes" to live a healthy and balanced life? Well, wonder no more—you do! Our memory verse this week reminds us that through God's divine power we have "everything we need" for life and godliness.

What does our memory verse say is the source of our provision?

by his power he has given use everything we need to live a Godley life

What did God do for us?

he Called use by his own Glory and goodness

Now, keep repeating this phrase as you take a long walk today: "I've got what it takes!" God's purpose for us is that we receive the divine power He has for us. He wants us to be strong, not weak. In what areas do you feel weak today?

_____

_____

_____

_____

_____

The power and strength of God lives within us by His Holy Spirit, and the revelation of that truth releases spiritual power in our lives that strengthens both our bodies and spirits. The Greek word *dunamis* is often used in reference to the power of the Holy Spirit available to us. This word is the root word of "dynamic," "dynamo" and "dynamite." Dynamite power, by way of the Holy Spirit, enables us to be dynamic witnesses, more than conquerors—spiritual dynamos—and stronger people.

Day 1 PRAY FOR POWER

Holy Spirit, dwell within me and grant me the dynamic power
that only You provide. In Christ's name, Amen.

Read Ephesians 3:14-21. Paul knew God's power in a personal way. He experienced it every day of his life, and testified to it when he wrote to the believers at Ephesus. He prayed that they, too, would receive this power. Write down verse 16, and substitute your name for the word "you."

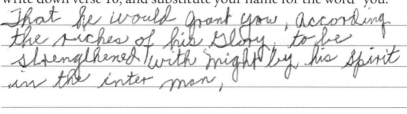

That he would grant you, according
the riches of his Glory, to be
strengthened with might by his Spirit
in the inter man,

_____

From where does the power come?

from the Holy Spirit,

And where does he pray you would receive such power?

that Christ may dwell in your hearts by faith that ye, being rooted and grounded in love,

Paul prays in verses 18 and 19 for power in you so that what things might result?

You may have *comperhend* to grasp how _____ . _____ and _____ and
_____ and _____ is the _____ of Christ,
and to _____ this _____ that surpasses all
knowledge—that you may be _____ to the measure of all the
_____ of God.

Love seems to be a key concept that God longs for us to understand in order to experience His full power. What is the hardest part for you of grasping God's unconditional love?

Paul closes his prayer for the Ephesians with a doxology that praises "the God who is able to do more than all we ask or imagine." Do you sometimes secretly feel your quest for a healthy weight or emotional healing is too much for God to accomplish? What would it take for you to believe that God can do even *more* than what you ask or imagine?

no, yes I believe that very thing. I know because, He He done it in my life throw faith and believing.

How does verse 20 say that God accomplishes these things for us?

now unto him that is able to do exceeding abundantly above all we ask or think according to the power of God, that worketh in use.

Have you prayed for God's divine power to fill your life so that you may fulfill God's purpose for you? Write a simple prayer here, closing with your own doxology of praise:

Yes I have prayed that prayer, And I pray it quite often.

Heavenly Father, help me remember today that nothing is impossible with You, even on my journey towards balanced health. In Christ's name, Amen.

Day 2 SOURCE OF POWER

Father, please help me when I'm tempted to go back to my old ways and try to accomplish goals through my own strength. In Christ's name, Amen.

Read Galatians 3:1-5. How do we daily tap into the Source of all power? By spending time in the Spirit's presence through daily spiritual disciplines that include prayer, a study of God's Word and meditation. Too often we either skip this aspect of our lives or fast-forward it and thus we move forward only in our own power. While we may be blessed with a certain amount of strength, we inevitably come to the end of our resources all too soon and then find ourselves "running on empty."

First Place 4 Health offers many resources to guide in proper nutrition through the Live It program. There is a good balance between protein and carbohydrates and good fats. Taken in proper doses, our bodies function more efficiently with the right foods in the right amounts. This is an amazing discovery for any former fast-food junkies used to piling on empty calories only to discover more hunger than satisfaction.

But some of us also suffer from being spiritual fast-food junkies. Our devotional lives have devolved into quickly checking in with God, reading a verse, tossing up a prayer and being on our way. Author Nancy Leigh DeMoss confessed such tendencies this way:

> I had allowed deadlines, projects, and demands to take priority over my relationship with the Lord. Oh, I still had a quiet time— of sorts. I usually managed to get in some sort of spiritual meal. But all too frequently, that meal had come to consist of hurriedly reading a short passage of scripture just before running out the door to accomplish one more thing for God. Spiritually, I was living in fast-food drive-throughs. I was having my devotions, if you could call it that. But I wasn't having devotion. I wasn't meeting with God. I wasn't nurturing our relationship.[1]

How can you move beyond "fast food" devotions to those that will nourish your soul? In Paul's letter to the Galatians, he chastises believers for "beginning with the Spirit" but then "trying to attain your goal by human effort."

As you think of your lifelong journey to better health, how would you describe your earlier efforts, before First Place 4 Health?

_____

_____

_____

_____

What about now? Do you find that you still have a tendency to rely on your willpower alone?

_____

_____

_____

_____

_____

What does Paul call folks who do such things (see v. 3)?

_____

_____

_____

_____

_____

What do you do when you want to grow a friendship?

_____

_____

_____

_____

_____

What parallels can you draw with growing your friendship/relationship with God?

_____

_____

_____

_____

_____

_____

Dearest Jesus, spending time with You is important and life-giving. May I always seek You first in my daily schedule. In Christ's name, Amen.

LIVE BY THE SPIRIT

*Help! I keep giving in to what my flesh wants and ignoring what
You want, Lord. Help me to resist temptations through the
power of the Holy Spirit. In Christ's name, Amen.*

God promises to give us His divine power every day. In fact, according to
Ephesians 5:18, we are filled afresh with the Holy Spirit daily. Write that
verse here:

_____

_____

_____

_____

_____

_____

In the New Testament Greek, that word "filled" actually implies that we
are to receive a continuous infilling, one that never stops. We never have
to run on empty! God's people are called to live continuously in the
power of the Holy Spirit. Easy to say, hard to do. Our natural tendency
is to live in the power of our own strength (or "the flesh"). Read Galatians 5:13-18. This passage is a reminder that Christ has set us free, but
that doesn't mean "free to go back to old ways." In verse 13 we are told:

Do not _____ ;

_____

rather, _____

_____

What is Paul's warning in verse 15?

_____

_____

_____

_____

What is the antidote to this kind of behavior (see v. 16)?

_____

_____

_____

_____

Using verse 17, describe what the sinful nature desires. What does the Spirit desire?

_____

_____

_____

_____

According to that verse, what is the result of this conflict?

_____

_____

_____

_____

_____

Almighty God, please forgive my sins—the times today I have chosen my way instead of Your way. In Christ's name, Amen.

Day 4 EMPOWERED FROM ABOVE

Lord, I do have faith but I'm not always sure how that should be manifested in my life. Show me, please. In Christ's name, Amen.

Read John 14:12-19. For many First Place 4 Health members, the hardest commitment to keep is daily exercise. Both mind and body often rebel at this activity, which is necessary for balanced living. Are we doomed to failure? No, God has given us everything we need—even to get these bodies moving, no matter what comes our way.

What are some of the promises Jesus makes in verses 12-14?

_____

_____

_____

_____

Which Person of the Trinity is promised to live within you (see vv. 16-17)?

_____

_____

_____

How does the Spirit fulfill in your life Christ's promise in verses 18-19?

_____

_____

_____

Exercising isn't just good for your body; it's good for your soul. Fitness instructor Theresa Rowe reminds us that it's important to nourish your mind, body and spirit: "The road to wellness is a journey, not a destination. Wake up fifteen minutes earlier and practice deep breathing exercises while you pray. And, remember, working out five to ten minutes a day is one hundred percent better than zero! It's never too late to start."[2] There are other benefits to being physically fit, including:

- It helps the body burn fat and protects against the muscle loss associated with low-calorie eating plans.
- It helps the body maintain or increase its metabolic rate; may help suppress appetite.
- It allows for weight loss on a higher calorie eating plan, which helps the body get all the nutrients it needs.
- It improves mood and self-esteem.

- It results in important health benefits such as lower blood pressure, improved cholesterol levels and increased fitness.
- It promotes long-term weight maintenance.

Have you asked God to help you exercise each day? If not, do so now in a short prayer.

_____

_____

_____

_____

Thank You, Lord, for getting me moving more each day and for helping me overcome any sedentary tendencies. In Christ's name, Amen.

Day 5 REFLECT GOD'S GLORY

Father, even though I don't feel I'm always a good model for the Christian life, please shine Your light through me. In Christ's name, Amen.

Read 2 Corinthians 3:17-18. Write two specific ways this verse encourages you today:

_____

_____

_____

_____

God's glory is manifested whenever He indwells a person and enables them to be or do what they could never be or do on their own. Thus divinely empowered, their accomplishments reflect the glory of God. Write of a time when your life brought glory to God. What happened?

_____

_____

_____

_____

In this passage of Paul's letter to the Corinthians, the apostle reminds us that it is through the Spirit's power that we are able to change our lives. What changes have you seen since you began this Bible study?

_____

_____

_____

_____

One young woman, Regina, knew all the right things to say but discovered she wasn't seeking better health for the right reasons; she needed to be "transformed into His likeness" (2 Corinthians 3:18).

"When I joined a Christian-based weight-loss program, I thought I had found the answer [to my search for self-worth]. I would silence the voices by finding the body I'd always wanted—and I would be pursuing God in the process. My motive, though, was wrong. I was joining the program not to become healthy but to be thin. I wasn't pursuing God so He could create a new heart in me; I was turning my weight loss over to God so He would create a new outward person for me to live in."[3]

In other words, her heart hadn't bought into the program. But God knows our hearts—He knows why we do what we do (including this Bible study today) and He does not condemn us. However, He *does* want to change our hearts.

Regina finally found freedom when she recognized that "I had asked God to change the way I looked, to help me diet, to help me exercise every day, to help me find the right clothes, to make me anyone but me. But in all my asking for solutions to my insecurities, I had never asked Him to change my heart."[4]

One of the reasons we often fail in pursuing weight management is that we neglect to address inner spiritual or emotional issues that have outer physical manifestations. Transformation ultimately comes from a total change of heart. Perhaps you began this journey with one goal in mind—for instance, to lose 25 pounds. But perhaps now you realize there is more involved in balanced healthy living than just numbers on a scale.

In what ways is God changing/transforming your heart?

_____

_____

_____

_____

Change my heart, O God. Make it ever new. Change my heart, O God.
May I be like You. In Christ's name, Amen.

Day
6

REFLECTION AND APPLICATION

Holy Spirit, I need You as my Counselor and my Guide. Amen.

Feeling powerless is debilitating and demoralizing. We want to do something, anything, to make something happen, but all too often we just
throw our hands up in the air and admit defeat. We feel powerless
against all odds. Health is an area where this occurs, often because we
feel at the mercy of our own bodies, which seem to rebel against us—even
when we're trying to do the right thing for them! That's why this week's
study is so important. We are *not* powerless—we have power from God
through the Holy Spirit. We can do what He calls us to do, not in our
own strength and will, but in partnership with Him.

Read John 14:25-27. What does Jesus call the Holy Spirit?

_____

_____

_____

What does He say about what the Holy Spirit will do in your life?

_____

_____

_____

_____

Jesus says that He leaves us with peace. When was the last time you experienced peace?

_____

_____

_____

_____

_____

Jesus points out that His peace is nothing like the peace we find in the world. His peace comes in the midst of chaos. It is the sense of wellbeing and full trust that, though the world around you is going crazy, God is still on the throne. He is in control. Be at peace.

The last part of verse 27 gives what admonition?

Do not _____

_____

and do not _____

_____

Why not take some time today to experience God's peace? It will mean withdrawing from your normal habitat (where everything around you calls out for attention) and being still before the Lord. Write down some words you associate with the concept of "peace."

_____

_____

_____

_____

_____

_____

Prince of Peace, will You come into my heart and fill me with a knowledge that You are in control and all is well? In Christ's name, Amen.

REFLECTION AND APPLICATION

Heavenly Father, I've been so distracted this week and pray You'll help me focus on things that truly matter. In Christ's name, Amen.

Today, why not try going a whole day unplugged—without all your technology! Don't answer your cell phone (unless it's an emergency, of course), don't check your email, don't log into Facebook or do a Twitter update. Be unavailable for a change and see how God will make His presence known to you in a new way.

If you chose to do this experiment, what did you notice about being "unplugged"?

_____

_____

_____

_____

_____

_____

_____

_____

Author Fil Anderson shares how he came to a point where he had to make some hard choices for turning off the world occasionally so that he could tune in to God:

> With pagers and cell phones, faxes and instant messaging, email and voice mail, streaming audio and video, the world is simply too much with us. . . . I could see the striking contrast between my empty life and the promise of a life of peace. I could see that each misfit part of my soul was sewn to the others with one common thread: distractions, keeping me from hearing the true voice of God. I was too distracted and consumed with activity to notice the quiet Voice. My deafness produced a life without peace.[5]

With your planner and your journal, make a plan for periodic times away when you can focus on God and your life. Start with an afternoon and perhaps work into one day a month for a quiet retreat. God will meet you there and fill you with His power.

Gracious God, may I be quiet long enough to hear Your voice and to respond in obedience and joy. In Christ's name, Amen.

Notes
1. Nancy Leigh DeMoss, *A Place of Quiet Rest* (Chicago, IL: Moody Publishers, 2000).
2. Theresa Rowe, "Soul Trainer," *Guideposts*, February 2009, p. 79.
3. Regina Franklin, *Who Calls Me Beautiful?* (Grand Rapids, MI: Discovery House Publishers, 2004), p. 39.
4. Ibid., p. 41.
5. Fil Anderson, *Running on Empty* (Colorado Springs, CO: NavPress, 2004) pp. 13,23.

Group Prayer Requests

4 first place
health

Today's Date: _____

Name	Request
Ann	Concerned wanters the anne results. Daughter had Crowens Custady arm God pertects her
Sue	before. Lost his Job & room Mate her dads going hospi. I am going to help my mother.
Tony	going to be Induced. Took her Cor & her purse
mae	
Linda	People pleaser. And learn to say no shes doing her tapes & lying about the information! she Cant do her tapes
Joy	Kens strounger thy gave him stranger Drugs. Infuestion for her magron
Tony	took her Car

Results

_____
_____
_____
_____
_____

look
inward

SCRIPTURE MEMORY VERSE
Search me, O God, and know my heart; test me and know my anxious thoughts. See if there is any offensive way in me, and lead me in the way everlasting.
PSALM 139:23-24

In this week's memory verse, King David asks God to enter the depths of his life—his heart—and to reveal his desires, actions, thoughts, habits, beliefs or sin. This is all to one purpose: so that David might then be led to the "way everlasting."

Any true search for God's purpose for our lives must include a time of looking inward. That can be really scary! Often, we expend lots of energy covering up and building walls of protection.

There are many coping mechanisms we can use to avoid facing ugly truths about ourselves—and emotional eating is one of them. Some of us have used food for comfort, love, security, companionship, distraction and as a way to numb ourselves so we wouldn't have to face the real issues that needed spiritual transformation. Our sin is not that we're overweight; it's that we turn to food (or any other substance or habit) to meet needs that only God can meet.

Ouch. Have your toes just been stepped on? Well, if they have, please know this: As we look inward this week, God is already there. He does not want to step on our toes; He wants to heal our hearts.

GOD KNOWS ME—INSIDE AND OUT

*God, it's a bit gritty inside my heart, but I know that You will help
me become clean and changed. In Christ's name, Amen.*

Do you believe you can hide from God? We may have everyone else
fooled about what we do or who we are, but God—our Creator and Re-
deemer—simply knows everything about us. Read Psalm 139:1-4,13-16.
What are the things King David observes in verses 1-4 about God and
what He knows?

_____

_____

_____

_____

How does it make you feel to acknowledge that God knows all about you?

_____

_____

_____

_____

What thoughts have you had lately that you wish God didn't know?
(Write these in your journal if you're concerned about privacy.)

_____

_____

_____

_____

In verses 13-16, we read of God's earliest knowledge of us and our bodies. Write down verse 14 here:

_____

_____

_____

_____

Do you praise God for your body, or are you more likely to blame Him?

_____

_____

_____

_____

What does it mean for you to acknowledge that God ordained all your days before you were even born (see v. 16)? (Yes, even *those* days . . .)

_____

_____

_____

_____

In response to life's wounds, sometimes people turn to behaviors that either release tension or numb pain. We've already mentioned emotional eating as one of those, but there are many other habits, such as gambling, workaholism, explosive anger, substance abuse or sexual impurity, that can become addictive. Pretty soon, such things take on a life of their own and begin to grip us so we can't stop ourselves. Unless we call on God to reveal in the light what we do in the dark, we can never address the root issues and come clean. Hiding such things only increases our shame and prevents the needed healing and hope-giving redemption.

Examine your heart and pray for God to search out what you need to address in your inner soul so that you may walk fully in the light of Christ. Compose your own version of our memory verse here:

_____

_____

_____

Thank You, Lord, for revealing even those hard things about my life, actions and choices. Let's work on them together. In Christ's name, Amen.

GOD'S LOVE CHANGES ME

*Gracious God, I cringe sometimes when I think of mistakes I have
made in the past. Thank You for being willing to love me into a new life.
In Christ's name, Amen.*

Have you heard that old joke, "The reality check is in the mail . . ."?
Reality is sometimes a jolt to the system, but facing the truth of what is
going on inside of us is a necessary first step toward any positive change.
Because God created us and loves us unconditionally, He wants us to be
whole and able to fulfill His purpose. Unfortunately, that usually comes
through change, which is hard. But change can also be life giving.

Read Ephesians 2:1-10. In verses 1-3, we see a picture of those who follow the ways of the world and of the enemy of our souls. How does Paul
describe that kind of life and behavior?

_____

_____

_____

_____

_____

How would you translate this to describe your behaviors before em-
barking on your First Place 4 Health journey?

_____

_____

_____

What did God do and why did He do it (see vv. 4-7)?

_____

_____

_____

_____

Write a prayer of thanks to God for His actions on your behalf.

_____

_____

_____

_____

_____

_____

If you fully understand and embrace the meaning in verses 8 and 9, your life will be changed forever. What does it mean to be "saved by grace through faith"?

_____

_____

_____

What about the phrases "the gift of God" and "so that no one can boast"?

_____

_____

_____

Have you ever tried to earn God's salvation—to be perfect and receive His love as a reward? What was the result?

_____

_____

_____

_____

In the book _Amazed by Grace,_ we read, "Grace is God giving us what we don't deserve; mercy is God not giving us what we do deserve. So the very nature of grace is that it is undeserved. To show grace is to extend favor to one who doesn't deserve it and can never earn it. But what do we deserve as a result of our sin and efforts to take God's place as controller of our lives? We deserve judgment and punishment. That's where both mercy and grace come in—God in His infinite mercy does not give us the death we deserve, but as an act of grace grants us forgiveness and new life."[1] That forgiveness and new life come when we place our faith in Him. Have you ever thought your works would get you into heaven (see v. 9)? If so, what do you believe now?

It is important to note that while our works don't earn us God's love, we are created for good works as a response to the love God has granted us as His children. As you read verse 10, write down ways you have been loved, forgiven and changed.

What are some of the works you believe God has created you to do?

Okay, Lord, I give up. I'm going to stop striving right now and rest in Your life-changing gifts of grace and mercy from now on. In Christ's name, Amen.

CONSEQUENCES OF BAD CHOICES
Day 3

Heavenly Father, I tried it my way and things got worse. I'm going to do it Your way from now on. In Christ's name, Amen.

Have you ever quipped something like this: "If I eat this cookie standing up (or in my bedroom or while driving), the calories don't count"? How ridiculous that sounds, and yet most of us discover when we record our daily intake on the Live It Tracker that we've fallen prey to a number of "lurking nibbles," while cooking, cleaning up, serving kids, and so on. The choices we make produce consequences. Good choices produce good results. Poor choices bring heartache and often failure. Paul reminds the Galatians that "we reap what we sow."

Read Galatians 6:7-8. Write down the life lesson revealed in verse 8.

The one who sows to please his sinful nature will reap _____.
The one who sows to please the Spirit will reap _____ _____.

Even though we know this life lesson is true, there seem to be little triggers that cause us to occasionally follow the path away from health and wholeness. When you have turned the wrong way in the past week, what has been the trigger(s)?

_____

_____

_____

_____

Singer Mandisa was a contestant on *American Idol* who was mocked by judge Simon Cowell due to her weight: "I think we're going to need a bigger stage." After forgiving him and testifying on network television, she was then voted off the reality show. Her health challenges had played out in public for everyone to see, and the ensuing letdown caused Mandisa to cry out to God:

I was standing up for You, and I was on that stage trying to proclaim how good You are. How could You let this happen to me? I dealt with my anger by eating: pizza, fast food, entire pies, Krispy Kreme donuts. I ate just about everything imaginable, and I was miserable. I was in the biggest pit of my life, and I shut everybody out. I turned the ringer off my phone. I didn't talk to the Lord.[2]

Fortunately, in the midst of this spiritual and emotional wilderness, God's unconditional love broke through to Mandisa and began a healing in her heart, which also jumpstarted a physical improvement and an 80-pound weight loss. Isn't it interesting to note that heart healing and body healing often go hand in hand? Mandisa continues:

I wish I'd sought God and turned to His Word and not shut out everybody who loves me and could have spoken godly wisdom into my life. I eventually learned the power of praising God when you don't feel like it. I think that's the most important time to worship the Lord because when you magnify Him, your problems look smaller by comparison. If I'd done that, I don't think I would have gotten into that pit. The next difficult situation I face, I'll know to turn to God, to look for His lessons and higher purposes and redemption.[3]

When one of your triggers threatens to turn you down the wrong path in the coming week, what are two things you can do to "turn to God, to look for His lessons and higher purposes and redemption"?

_____

_____

_____

_____

Thank You for continuing to put people in my path who help to turn me back to You and who speak truth into my soul. In Christ's name, Amen.

HIDDEN THOUGHTS

Dear Heavenly Father, I know that You search my motives and my desires, and I ask that You would help me to grow today in godliness. In Christ's name, Amen.

As we ask God to look within us, we must pray that He will give us the mind of Christ. Most battles begin and end in the mind—the body and actions simply follow our intellectual choices. Have you asked God to search your thoughts? Are you enslaved to negativity or a spirit of defeat? Read 1 Corinthians 2:10-16. In verses 10-12, how does Paul say that we can know the thoughts of God?

_____

_____

_____

_____

_____

In verses 13-16, we read about spiritual understanding on a deep level. How do you feel that God is granting you more discernment as you make daily choices to obey His Spirit?

_____

_____

_____

_____

_____

What practices can you do to help you keep your thoughts pure, positive and prayerful?

_____

_____

_____

_____

_____

Corrie ten Boom and her Christian family hid Jews in their Dutch home during World War II and were sent to concentration camps in punishment. Her family died, but Corrie emerged at the end of the war, vowing to be a "tramp for the Lord" and travel all over the world speaking of God's faithfulness and the power of forgiveness. Yet even this godly woman knew about the struggle with sin:

> If we look within ourselves we are bound to find more and more sin. . . . Why not pray with the psalmist, "Search me, O God, and know my heart." He will show you your sins. Not all of them at once, but increasingly you will recognize them, and always in the light of Christ's finished work upon the cross. Then God makes it very clear where you have to make restitution, and so you get right with God and right with men. To the end of our lives it remains a struggle against sin, but a victorious struggle. If only we put on the whole armor of God, we go from victory to victory.[4]

As God shows you the depths of your heart, are you discovering areas that need to be made right? What do you need to "get right with God and right with men"?

_____

_____

_____

_____

From whom do you need forgiveness today? How will you do that?

_____

_____

_____

Thank You, Lord, for giving me a mind that can think and reason and make godly choices. In Christ's name, Amen.

ENTER GOD'S PRESENCE

*Lord, I come to You now and seek Your guidance and grace for all that is
ahead of me on this new day. In Christ's name, Amen.*

Read Hebrews 10:19-25. The best way to grow in spirit is to consciously
enter into God's presence on an ongoing daily basis. How are we to draw
near to God (see v. 22)?

_____

_____

_____

_____

Which of these is hardest for you to do?

_____

_____

_____

_____

In God's presence, we're encouraged to do four important things (vv. 23-
25). List them here:

Let us _____

Let us _____

Let us _____

Let us _____

Someone once said we literally "spend" our lives, in a way similar to
spending money. Like a bank account, if we take continual withdrawals
and don't make deposits, we quickly become overdrawn. Author Nancie
Carmichael laments, "Over the years, I had not made the necessary 'deposits'—I had been running in the red, emotionally and physically for
too long. . . . The needs seemed so great, never ending. And yet I missed

a step—unless I received spiritual nourishment, there was no way I could continue to 'feed' others."[5]

Review the four activities we should engage in while in God's presence (vv. 23-25), and then write down one specific way you will pursue each one this week:

Hold on to hope _____

Spur one another _____

Meet together _____

Encourage one another _____

Gracious God, guide me to someone today who needs encouragement and a word from You. In Christ's name, Amen.

Day 6 REFLECTION AND APPLICATION

Father, I want to be beautiful, both inside and out. Please help me to work on both in a balanced manner. In Christ's name, Amen.

Read 1 Peter 3:3-4. As this week's study draws to a close, let's look at beauty—specifically, *inner* beauty. People today still mock inner beauty as though it were a poor runner-up to outer beauty. In fact, there's even a reality television show based on that premise. Yet God (the One who thought up beauty in the first place!) says that inner beauty is the winner, not the consolation prize. This passage from Peter states what is of great worth in God's sight.

Describe that beauty (see v. 4).

_____

_____

_____

_____

Do you know people with a gentle and quiet spirit? How does being in their presence make you feel?

_____

_____

_____

_____

What do you think you'd have to do to display those qualities?

_____

_____

_____

_____

Read 1 Samuel 16:7. In this story, God tells Samuel, who is searching for Israel's next king, how His ways are in contrast to the world's ways. How do you formulate a first impression of someone? What do you notice first?

_____

_____

_____

_____

When evaluating a person, what does God see first and foremost?

_____

_____

_____

_____

What our culture values is displayed at every turn in the media, advertisements, celebrities and pop culture. But these are faulty mirrors. When we look into them, all they point out is what we lack. In order to move into wholeness and discover God's purpose for our lives, we need to consult different mirrors: reflections of what God says is true and holy through His Word, the Bible.

Who are two or three godly men or women who will be models to you of beauty?

_____

_____

_____

_____

God, give me a beautiful heart and may that be visible to all around me.
In Christ's name, Amen.

Day 7

REFLECTION AND APPLICATION

Father, this self-examination stuff can really be heavy, so I thank You
for reminding me of Your unconditional love for me in the process.
In Christ's name, Amen.

As you have looked inward this week, perhaps you have discovered some things God wants to reveal to you along your journey to a more balanced life—physically, emotionally, spiritually and mentally. Look over your notes from this week and jot down one lesson learned from each day's study:

Day 1: "God Knows Me—Inside and Out"

_____

_____

_____

Day 2: "God's Love Changes Me"

_____

_____

_____

Day 3: "Consequences of Bad Choices"

_____

_____

_____

_____

Day 4: "Hidden Thoughts"

_____

_____

_____

_____

Day 5: "Enter God's Presence"

_____

_____

_____

_____

Day 6: "Inner Beauty"

_____

_____

_____

_____

Perhaps the most important takeaway is to realize that God wants to use us, no matter what has happened (or not happened) in our past. He can make us new creatures and fulfill His purpose for us, despite our mistakes and poor choices. Does this give you hope? Write down a dream you have, a dream that can only happen through the power and promise of God:

_____

_____

_____

_____

Commit this dream to the Lord and ask Him to show you each step necessary toward fulfilling His purpose for your life. Finally, take a look at
men and women of the Bible whom God used in spite of their past:

Abraham, founder of Israel and tagged "the friend of God," was
once a worshipper of idols. Joseph had a prison record but later
became prime minister of Egypt. Moses was a murderer, but later
became the one who delivered his nation from the slavery of
Pharaoh. Jephthah was an illegitimate child who ran around
with a tough bunch of hoods before he was chosen by God to
become His personal representative.

Rahab was a harlot in the streets of Jericho but was later
used in such a mighty way that God enlisted her among the
members of His hall of fame in Hebrews 11. Eli and Samuel were
both poor, inconsistent fathers, but proved to be strong men in
God's hand regardless. Jonah and John Mark were missionaries
who ran away from hardship like cowards but were ever-so-
profitable later on.

Peter openly denied the Lord and cursed Him, only to return
and become God's choicest spokesman among the early years of
the infant church. Paul was so hard and vicious in his early life
the disciples and apostles refused to believe he'd actually become
a Christian . . . but you know how greatly God used him. . . .

The files of heaven are filled with stories of redeemed, refit-
ted renegades and rebels. . . . God is not only willing but pleased
to use any vessel—just as long as it is clean today. It may be
cracked or chipped. It may be worn or it may have never been
used before. You can count on this—the past ended one second
ago. From this point onward, you can be clean, filled with His
Spirit, and used in many different ways for His honor.[6]

Below or in your journal, reflect on your past. Is there something in your
history that you don't believe God can redeem? If so, read the passage

above again and write a prayer, asking God to give you faith to believe in His power to use you, no matter your past.

_____

_____

_____

_____

_____

_____

_____

How humbled I am, heavenly Father, that You choose to use me in spite of all You know about me! In Christ's name, Amen.

Notes

1. Lucinda Secrest McDowell, *Amazed by Grace* (Bolivar, MO: Quiet Waters Publications, 2002), p. 23.
2. Camerin Courtney, "TCW Talks to Mandisa," *Today's Christian Woman*, July/August 2009, p. 19.
3. Ibid.
4. Corrie Ten Boom, *Not Good If Detached* (Fort Washington, PA: Christian Literature Crusade, 1957), p. 108.
5. Nancie Carmichael, *Praying for Rain* (Nashville, TN: Thomas Nelson Publishers, 2001), p. 61.
6. Charles Swindoll, *Growing Strong in the Seasons of Life* (Portland OR: Multnomah Press, 1983), pp. 373-374.

Group Prayer Requests

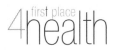

Today's Date: _____

Name	Request
Aquina	The baby has pneumonia
Tony	
Stacy	go to Christofer
Linda	she would fell better
Joy	Brenda give her favor with each place she has to go, for Ken.
Sue	meadater

Results

_____

_____

_____

_____

_____

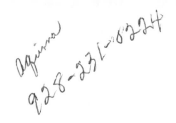

overcome
obstacles

SCRIPTURE MEMORY VERSE

Everyone born of God overcomes the world. This is the victory that has overcome the world, even our faith. Who is it that overcomes the world? Only he who believes that Jesus is the Son of God.

1 JOHN 5:4-5

What do you think of when you hear a person referred to as an "overcomer"? Chances are, you're reminded of someone who has faced major obstacles or catastrophic challenges, yet has persevered and been successful, prevailing against all odds.

According to verse 5 of our memory verse, who is an overcomer?

every one thats Born of God over Comes the World.

Are you born of God? Do you believe that Jesus is the Son of God? If so, are you an overcomer?

yes I am an over Comer

Write down the challenges that you are facing this week that you desire to overcome.

_____

_____

_____

_____

Day 1 | STRUGGLING INSIDE

Almighty God, this whole balanced life thing is a lot harder than I thought, so I'm glad You're not giving up on me. In Christ's name, Amen.

Sometimes we are our own worst enemy. We struggle against ourselves and our wills. We know what to do, yet we don't do it. When was the last time you experienced that inner struggle?

_____

_____

_____

_____

Read Romans 7:14-25. Does it surprise you to discover that even the apostle Paul wrestled in a similar way? What does Paul confess in verse 15?

_____

_____

_____

_____

_____

What does he identify as the source of his struggle (see vv. 17-20)?

_____

_____

_____

_____

What basic conclusion does he reach in verse 21?

I find Then a law that When I would for good, Evil is present with me.

Verses 22 and 23 describe how we can know what God wants—and even *want* what God wants—but still do the opposite. What is Paul's explanation for this behavior?

I delight in the Lord, after the inward man.

How are your body's desires at odds with your spirit's desires?

Write down where you can find rescue (see v. 25).

Joanna Weaver, author of *Having a Mary Spirit*, refers to the struggles Paul mentions as her battle with the part of herself she calls "Flesh Woman":

> Flesh Woman is that contrary, rebellious, incredibly self-centered version of you who shows up when things don't go the way you planned and life seems habitually unfair. . . . [She's the] righteous indignation we use to justify our not-so-righteous anger.

The flattery we pour on in order to secure coveted positions. The false humility in which we cloak ourselves while secretly hoping to be admired. Unfortunately, we rarely pause to wonder if what we're doing is wrong. And that's just where Flesh Woman wants it to be. For if you were to pull off her mask, you'd know what she's really up to. Her main goal is not your benefit, but her power base. Though Flesh Woman would never admit it, she's determined to do whatever it takes to remain in control of your life.[1]

Do you feel imprisoned by "Flesh Woman" or "Flesh Man"? Write a prayer, asking God to free you to obey Him.

_____

_____

_____

_____

Thank You, Lord, that You are in control and You will help me to be an overcomer. In Christ's name, Amen.

Day 2 — GOD'S COMFORT

Heavenly Father, Your presence and peace in the midst of my pain are a great comfort to me. In Christ's name, Amen.

It's hard to be in the middle of a fight for your life, isn't it? And yet, that's just what we feel like sometimes—that we are struggling just to keep our heads above water. One way that God enables us to become overcomers is through His presence and power. When Jesus calls the Holy Spirit "the Comforter," He is saying that the Spirit is our strength—His strength is what brings comfort to us. The word "comforter" as applied to the Holy Spirit in the original Greek is *paracleto*, which means "helper," "advocate" and "strengthener." Christ promised that this Strengthener would be with us forever.

Read 2 Corinthians 1:3-6. What names does Paul call God in verse 3?

_____

_____

_____

What does God do for us, and why does He do it (see v. 4)?

_____

_____

_____

Paul said two related things flow over our lives. What are they (see v. 5)?

_____

_____

_____

What does God's comfort achieve for a person who is seeking to be an overcomer (see v. 6)?

_____

_____

_____

Today is a good day to extend comfort to someone who needs it. Think of ways others have comforted you, and do the same to comfort someone else today. Who? Ask God to reveal a name to you as you go through your prayer list, read your church bulletin or even drive in your neighborhood. As you serve, you may find yourself comforted in the process.

Dearest Jesus, help me know who to comfort today and give me the boldness to reach out to them in Your name. In Christ's name, Amen.

ADOPTED BY GOD

Abba, thank You for adopting me into Your family so that I don't have to live as an orphan anymore. In Christ's name, Amen.

Read Romans 8:9-17. According to verses 15-17, what does it mean to be adopted by God?

_____

_____

_____

_____

_____

After participating in several adoptions, one Seattle attorney said, "I have begun to see in the lives of the adoptive families I work with a picture of God's love—for others and for me. I have concluded that recovering a biblical theology of adoption can help us know more about God and experience Him in new and vital ways."[2]

In verses 9-13, Paul reminds the Romans that they are controlled by the Spirit living in them. Write down each reference to what the Spirit does in those five verses.

_____

_____

_____

_____

_____

What is the end result? (The last three words of verse 13 have the answer.)

_____

_____

_____

_____

_____

In verse 14, Paul introduces a revolutionary concept that those who are led by the Spirit are _____ of God. What does that mean for us as it relates to fear (see v. 15)?

_____

_____

_____

_____

Abba is the Aramaic term for "Daddy." By suggesting that believers call the Creator of the Universe "Daddy," Paul is proposing a radical acknowledgement of intimate relationship with Him. Do you live in a "spirit of fear" or a "spirit of sonship" when it comes to your relationship to God? Explain.

_____

_____

_____

_____

When someone chooses to adopt a son or a daughter, a legal contract provides for a brand-new birth certificate, which states their relationship as parent and child from now on. That's a picture of what happened when we chose to become Christ-followers. How is this reality confirmed (see v. 16)?

_____

_____

_____

_____

And what will be the outcome (see v. 17)?

_____

_____

_____

_____

Write a prayer to your heavenly Father, sharing your feelings about being His adopted son or daughter.

Dear Abba,

_____

_____

_____

_____

_____

_____

Love, Your son/daughter, _____

I promise, heavenly Father, to live from now on as a daughter/son of the King of kings and Lord of lords! In Christ's name, Amen.

Day 4

MORE THAN CONQUERORS

Dear God, Your followers can do this together—we can conquer anything that comes our way and threatens to keep us from Your purpose. Amen.

More than conquerors. This was the theme at a recent banquet in Boston for the Joni and Friends ministry to the disabled. Joni Eareckson Tada was only 17 years old when she dove into a shallow pool and emerged a quadriplegic. Faced with numerous opportunities to give up in defeat, Joni has instead fought valiantly for more than 40 years—not only for her own life's meaning and ministry, but for the rights and the quality of both physical and spiritual lives of countless unnamed others who struggle against tremendous odds through their disabilities.

Joni would likely be the first to echo the apostle Paul: "No, in all these things we are more than conquerors through Him who loved us." We can all be overcomers if we realize that even in hard times, God is conforming us to His image.

Read Romans 8:35-39. Name seven specific things that threaten to separate you from Christ's love (see v. 35).

1. _____
2. _____
3. _____
4. _____
5. _____
6. _____
7. _____

Can they? Write down verse 37 as your answer.

_____
_____
_____
_____

In verses 38 and 39, Paul lists 10 more things that cannot separate us from Christ's love. List them here:

1. _____
2. _____
3. _____
4. _____
5. _____
6. _____
7. _____
8. _____
9. _____
10. _____

Joni Eareckson Tada says, "Sometimes God will use suffering and affliction to sandblast us to the core and get us seriously thinking about larger than life issues of heaven and hell. I just don't know that we would think about these issues if it were not for an ice-cold splash of suffering waking us out of our spiritual slumber. God's purpose in redeeming us is not to make our lives happy, healthy and free of trouble. It is not an escape from our physical pains. His purpose is to make us more like Christ. He will choose to allow spinal cord injury or multiple sclerosis or blindness or stroke or Alzheimer's or whatever to not only teach us, but also our loved ones, about what it means to become more like Him." What is God using in your life to teach you "what it means to become more like Him"?

_____

_____

_____

_____

Thank You, Lord, that literally nothing that comes my way can ever come between You and me—I'm counting on it! In Christ's name, Amen.

Day 5

WORTHY WEAPONS

Almighty God, may I be brave and wise enough to use the weapons You have provided as I seek to change my life. In Christ's name, Amen.

Read 2 Corinthians 10:1-6. Those of us who desire to become spiritual overcomers must realize that we do not live by the same standards as the world. In these verses, Paul contrasts "the world" with the life of a believer in several ways (see vv. 3-4). Explain what he means in your own words.

_____

_____

_____

_____

What are three ways we use God's weapons (see vv. 5-6)?

_____

_____

_____

One of the most important weapons in our arsenal is prayer. In fact, the Lord's Prayer ends with the plea for God to "deliver us from evil." And since there's evil around us at every turn, it's a good idea to pray the Lord's Prayer every single day! Prayer is a weapon that demolishes strongholds. If you are dealing with strongholds in your life (and who isn't?), perhaps the following prayer from Peter Scazzero's book *Daily Office* will help:

> Lord, You are right that I have a powerful demonic enemy seeking to lure me into a pit and dominate me. Snatch me from the evil one! Rescue me from Satan's desire to destroy my faith. Help me discern the temptations of Satan coming at me. Teach me to wait on You when tempted in the wilderness, like Jesus. I place my confidence in You, Father, to care for me today. You speak the truth when You say: "The one who is in you is greater than the one who is in the world" (1 John 4:4). So I affirm with King David: "I will not fear the tens of thousands drawn up against me on every side" (Psalm 3:6). You are good and Your love endures forever. Amen.[3]

When I am weak, Lord, You are strong. When I am afraid, Lord, You are brave for me. Thank You. In Christ's name, Amen.

REFLECTION AND APPLICATION

Day
6

Dear God of a thousand new beginnings, I'm grateful that You have offered me a fresh start at a life that is healthier on all levels. Amen.

Read 2 Corinthians 5:16-21. What does verse 17 mean to you, for your life?

_____

_____

_____

_____

_____

Look up the meaning of the word "reconciliation" and write it here:

_____

_____

_____

_____

What do you think Paul means when he writes of reconciliation in the following verses?

Reconciling us to God through Christ (v. 18):

_____

_____

_____

Giving us ministry of reconciliation (v. 18):

_____

_____

_____

God reconciling the world to Himself (v. 19):

_____

_____

_____

Committing us to the ministry of reconciliation (v. 19):

_____

_____

_____

Be reconciled to God (v. 20):

_____

_____

_____

_____

Do you see yourself as "Christ's ambassador" to the world (see v. 20)? How are you carrying out that role?

_____

_____

_____

If God's Son, Jesus, was perfect and sinless, why did He die on the cross (see v. 21)?

_____

_____

_____

If Jesus paid that ultimate price—death for our sins—then how do you think we should respond to Him, in our lives (see v. 21)?

_____

_____

_____

It may be hard to think of yourself as _righteous_. Perhaps it's a bit easier to think of yourself as _new_. In this newness of life, you can seek to live in a way that glorifies God and that seeks holiness.

Lord, sometimes when we're new, we don't always know how to act and what to do, but we thank You that You will show us the new path. Amen.

REFLECTION AND APPLICATION

*Lord, I give up. I give up all my own need to control circumstances
and people and yes, even You. In Christ's name, Amen.*

This week we have talked once again about how hard it can be to live a
life of faith and faithfulness. Yet, as we appropriate all God has for us, we
can truly be overcomers. Reflect on the week and try to write down one
gem of knowledge or encouragement from each day's study.

Day 1: "Struggling Inside":

_____

_____

_____

Day 2: "God's Comfort":

_____

_____

_____

Day 3: "Adopted by God":

_____

_____

_____

Day 4: "More than Conquerors":

_____

_____

_____

Day 5: "Worthy Weapons":

_____

_____

_____

Day 6: "New":

_____

_____

_____

One profound truth held by First Place 4 Health sounds like a strange formula for success: *If you want to live a balanced life—spiritually, mentally, emotionally and physically—start on your knees.* Carole Lewis reminds us that the idea of surrender isn't usually seen as a positive thing:

> We're not typically encouraged to surrender to anything or anybody. Surrender is what losing armies do. Surrender connotes the idea of weakness or loss. When we surrender it feels like we're losing control—perhaps even losing our identity. . . . What does surrender to the Lord look like? It starts by beginning every day with a simple thought and prayer: God, this day is for You. Every day is a new beginning, a new opportunity to dedicate ourselves and our actions to the Lord. Just start there—God, this day is for You. God will show you what to do next.[4]

Make time today to do a prayer walk. As you get into a good walking rhythm, try praying Carole's prayer: *God, this day is for You. God, this day is for You.* When you return from your adventure, take a few minutes to write in your journal about what God revealed on your journey together.

God, this day is for You. I dedicate myself to live as You purpose from now on, in Your power and strength. In Christ's name, Amen.

Notes

1. Joanna Weaver, *Having a Mary Spirit* (Colorado Springs, CO: WaterBrook, 2006), p. 12.
2. David V. Andersen, "When God Adopts," *Christianity Today*, July 9, 1993, p. 36.
3. Peter Scazzero, *Daily Office* (Elmhurst, NY: Emotionally Healthy Spirituality, 2008), p. 163.
4. Carole Lewis, *First Place 4 Health* (Ventura, CA: Gospel Light, 2008), p. 93.

Group Prayer Requests

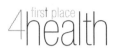

Today's Date: _____

Name	Request

Results

_____

_____

_____

_____

_____

_____

listen to
God's voice

SCRIPTURE MEMORY VERSE

*Whether you turn to the right or to the left, your ears will hear
a voice behind you, saying, "This is the way; walk in it."*

ISAIAH 30:21

Mike got what he wanted for Christmas: a GPS—global positioning system. He was thrilled. Now he could program any address, stick the small unit on the dashboard of his car and follow the GPS's voice instructions directly to his destination!

But first he had to choose a voice. There were at least four options: American accented male or female, or British accented male or female. He decided on the British female voice and promptly named "her" Guinevere Penelope Simonington (GPS).

From then on, whatever Guinevere Penelope said in that hoity-toity voice, Mike did to the nth degree. Except that sometimes, Guinevere Penelope gave instructions that were a wee bit off the mark. When that happened, Mike would go his own way, giving GPS time to reconfigure and catch up with him. Once when one of Mike's passengers wryly observed this behavior and said, "So, what good is it to have GPS if you still have to figure out whether or not to do what she says?"

Exactly. Either we listen to the voice and obey, or we listen to the voice, think about what we want to do on our own and obey only as we see fit. Sometimes obedience suits us, sometimes not. Aren't we a bit like that with God? On one hand, we certainly want Him to give us explicit directions and guidance in all things. But sometimes we are convinced that what He says must be a little "off," so we decide to go our way after all and let Him catch up, redirecting all the while . . .

Day 1 — GOD ANSWERS

Father, please help me to hear Your voice and Your answer
amidst the cacophony of the world today. In Christ's name, Amen.

Read Isaiah 30:1-23. Isaiah 30 is an entire chapter about how God keeps telling Israel what they need to do in order to be delivered from their enemies. But they simply do not want to hear and obey—they continue to wallow in the consequences of their actions. These "chosen people" have rebelled against God and sought negotiations with Egypt. But God still doesn't give up on them.

What three items of good news does Isaiah give the Israelites in verse 19?

1. *Thou Shell weep no more*
2. *he shell will be very gracious*
3. *at the voce of your cry the will answer*

List the two negatives and two positives found in verse 20.

give you the bread of adversity
And the water of Affection
yet the the teachers Shell not be moved in Corner no more, But thy eyes shell see the teachers

Think about your life recently and write down some experiences of:

The bread of adversity

_____

_____

_____

The water of affliction

_____
_____
_____

When God's voice makes your path clear (as stated in verse 21), what should be your response? Follow the Israelites' example in verse 22 to guide you in thinking of specific actions to take. What could be some modern-day equivalents to their response to God?

you lesson to What hes
_____
_____
_____
_____

Has anything or anyone become an idol in your life? Explain.

_____
_____
_____
_____
_____

Verse 23 elaborates further on God's gracious provision. What does this mean to you in your present circumstances?

_____
_____
_____
_____
_____

Gracious God, I know I need to lay down all the idols that have taken precedence over You in my life. Today I name them before You and leave them at your feet. In Christ's name, Amen.

Day 2

EARS WIDE OPEN

Father, I'm going to try to speak less and listen more today.
Starting now. In Christ's name, Amen.

Yes, it's true that God gave us two ears and only one mouth for a reason. And yet, some days our mouth is open far more often than our ears. In order to truly listen to God's voice, we must have our ears and our heart wide open. Read Proverbs 23:12. What is King Solomon's advice?

_____

_____

_____

_____

Name one instruction you have received recently in your First Place 4 Health group that you need to apply to your heart.

_____

_____

_____

_____

British professor and author C. S. Lewis once referred to pain as "God's megaphone." Sometimes God has to shout at us to get our attention. And, sometimes, pain is the very thing that does it.

When Billy and Ruth Graham's home was being built in Montreat, North Carolina, Ruth was on the construction site speaking with one of the carpenters. Engrossed in conversation, she leaned against a piece of equipment and promptly heard a harsh shout from another worker. As she recoiled, he apologized, "I'm so sorry, Mrs. Graham, but you were about to lose your fingers!" Ruth had been leaning next to a moving saw blade. She wisely observed, "I will always be grateful to that man for yelling at me."

Write down a time when an experience of pain or suffering redirected your attention back to God and spiritual matters.

_____

_____

_____

_____

_____

Did that incident force you to turn to God more and listen to His voice, or did you return to your former ways once the crisis was past?

_____

_____

_____

_____

_____

Gracious God, I didn't much like it when You "shouted" at me through that hard experience, but it did teach me something. Thank You. Amen.

OTHER LOUD VOICES

Day 3

Father, I've had all kinds of video tapes playing in my mind for years and ask You to erase them so I can hear and see the truth from You. Amen.

In her book *Who Calls Me Beautiful?* Regina Franklin states the following about identifying the "other voices" that speak into our lives:

We must learn to identify the words spoken by the one who seeks to destroy our souls. Satan is a liar. Deception is at the core of his being. We must identify his words when we hear them—words of rejection, hatred, failure and discontent:
   "I'll never measure up."
   "I can never be beautiful."

"If I were prettier, people would love me."

"I'm not good at anything."

"If I had new clothes, I'd be satisfied with the way I look."

"I'm so fat."

All lies. Words of death, not life. If he can convince us that we're worthless, he can immobilize us and keep us from fulfilling God's plan in our lives. Out of fear of rejection we won't reach out to others. We'll wallow in self-hatred. Out of fear of failure, we won't follow our dreams. We'll drown in discontent.[1]

Yesterday's reading suggested that we apply our ears to knowledge—but that can be easier said than done. Today there are numerous voices that tickle our ears on any subject. You can probably find an argument that defends just about any course of action. You can definitely find countless diets and get-thin-quick schemes. Everyone has a gimmick and an angle. So how do you know which voice is true?

Read Isaiah 8:19-23. Isaiah addresses this very dilemma in verses 19-20. What does he say to do?

_____

_____

_____

_____

_____

_____

What is the penalty for heeding the wrong voices (see vv. 21-22)?

_____

_____

_____

_____

_____

_____

Have you ever lashed out at God after you listened to the wrong voices and got burned?

_____

_____

_____

_____

_____

In his book *Emotionally Healthy Spirituality,* Pastor Peter Scazzero states that voices of the surrounding world and our pasts often repeat the deeply held negative beliefs we may have learned in our families and cultures growing up, such as:

- ❏ I am a mistake.
- ❏ I am a burden.
- ❏ I am stupid.
- ❏ I am worthless.
- ❏ I am not allowed to make mistakes.
- ❏ I must be approved by certain people to feel okay.
- ❏ I don't have the right to experience joy and pleasure.
- ❏ I don't have the right to assert myself and say what I think and feel.
- ❏ I don't have a right to feel.
- ❏ I am valued based on my intelligence, wealth, and what I do, not for who I am.[2]

Put a check by any of these negative phrases that have ever reflected your own beliefs, and then explain why you checked those here:

_____

_____

_____

_____

_____

Peter Scazzero goes on to state that if we can embrace the fact that we are unconditionally loved by God, we can instead embrace a more biblical self-understanding as reflected in these statements:

☐ I hold myself in high regard despite my imperfections and limits.
☐ I am worthy to assert my God-given power in the world.
☐ I am entitled to exist.
☐ It is good that I exist.
☐ I have my own identity from God that is distinct and unique.
☐ I am worthy of being valued and paid attention to.
☐ I am entitled to joy and pleasure.
☐ I am entitled to make mistakes and not be perfect.[3]

Put a check by at least three of these positive phrases that you want to embrace in your life this week. Explain why you're choosing those three here:

_____

_____

_____

_____

Help me, heavenly Father, to remember that Your voice is the One who speaks truth into my life and all others must be carefully screened through Your Word. In Christ's name, Amen.

Day
4

LISTEN UP!

Lord, You know that I would often rather give advice than take it, but I'm trying hard to change and I appreciate You helping me do just that. In Christ's name, Amen.

Do you like to take advice? Or are you one of those folk who love to dole out opinions to others, but rarely heed the advice someone offers you? King Solomon (the wisest man in the world, by the way) equates wisdom with listening to advice in both Proverbs 12 and 13. According to Proverbs 12:15, what is the difference between a fool and a wise person?

_____

_____

_____

_____

To whom do you most often go for advice? What is usually the outcome?

_____

_____

_____

Read Proverbs 13:10. Do you think pride plays a part in your decision whether or not to take godly counsel? What are the consequences of pride, according to this verse?

_____

_____

_____

_____

What factors do you use to determine whose advice to heed?

_____

_____

_____

_____

In *The Echo Within,* author Robert Benson advises:

> Sometimes people hesitate to give God any credit for being able to work through the ordinary of our lives, through the very sentences we hear and say. Such touchstone sentences are affirmations, not commands; they illumine rather than instruct. They

help you get your bearings, but they do not offer marching orders. . . . They do not say where you are going next as much as they reinforce the direction in which you are heading. To the degree they point you toward a new road, it will most always be a new road with which you are already familiar.[4]

In what "ordinary ways" is God speaking into your life this week?

_____

_____

_____

_____

*Thank You, Father, for using good voices of truth to help guide me
and show me Your purpose for my life. In Christ's name, Amen.*

Day
5

GOD SPEAKS THROUGH HIS WORD

*Gracious God, thank You for the Bible and the way it is coming alive as I
seek to know what You mean through Your Word. In Christ's name, Amen.*

Read 2 Timothy 3:16. What do you think Paul means when he writes that all Scripture is "God-breathed"?

_____

_____

_____

_____

If the Bible is truly God's Word, how does it seek to "speak" to each one of us?

_____

_____

_____

_____

Briefly describe your relationship with your Bible before you began working through *God's Purpose for You*.

_____

_____

_____

_____

And now? What, if anything, has changed?

_____

_____

_____

_____

The divinely inspired Scripture is useful for what four practices (see v. 16)?

1. _____

2. _____

3. _____

4. _____

Even after losing weight, Christian singer Mandisa admits that battling food addiction is the most difficult part of her weight-loss journey. Here's another story from her about how knowing Scripture guides her spiritual journey:

> I'm learning to replace the negative messages I picked up about my body with the truth of God's Word and what He says about me: that He loves me unconditionally and that I'm fearfully and wonderfully made. . . . But since I've been dealing with this addiction for 20 years, I'm not going to retrain my mind overnight. But thankfully God's Word is powerful. I've memorized a lot of scripture, and I've written many more verses on note cards. I used to travel with Beth Moore on her praise team and she'd always

say that on the eighth day God created note cards. She'd put scripture prayers on those cards, and now that's what I do. They're with me all the time.[5]

What are three things you can do to become more familiar with your own Bible?

_____

_____

_____

_____

_____

Almighty God, I remembered my verse today and it was just what I needed to know for the moment. Thanks. In Christ's name, Amen.

Day 6

REFLECTION AND APPLICATION

Dear God, You truly take me by Your hand and show me the path of life, and I praise You forever! In Christ's name, Amen.

Read Psalm 16:7-11. We can rest in God's truth. Today's Scripture passage is for you to use as a catalyst for praise and prayer to the God who speaks and "makes known to [you] the path of life." There are two particular things that God does, for which the psalmist gives praise in verse 7. What are they?

_____

_____

_____

_____

_____

One of the hard but good truths in life is that people are created with limits. But our bodies can "rest secure" (v. 9). We have limits, but our

God is unlimited! Write some of the benefits we receive from this limitless God. Use today's verses for inspiration.

_____

_____

_____

_____

_____

Medical doctor Richard Swenson speaks to the concern that people (including believers) have increasingly become overloaded:

> Since God is the author and creator of my limits, then it's probably okay with Him that I have limits. He probably does not expect me to be infinite and is a little surprised when I try. It is okay with Him if I am not all things to all people all the time all by myself. As a matter of fact, it is probably not okay with Him if I assume otherwise.
>
> You see, it's okay for me to have limits—God doesn't.
>
> It is okay for me to get a good night's sleep—God doesn't sleep.
>
> It is okay for me to rest—God doesn't need to.
>
> It is probably even okay to be depressed—because God isn't.
>
> We do not know a lot about what heaven looks like, but this much we know: God is not pacing the throne room anxious and depressed because of the condition of the world. He knows, He is not surprised, and He is sovereign.
>
> It's okay if we have limits. He is able.
>
> Limits were God's intention from the beginning. He decided early on that limits were not only good but necessary. It was His way of preempting any ambiguity about who is God and who is not. He is the Creator—the One without limits. We are the created—the ones with limits. . . . As the author of limits, God put them within us for our protection. We violate them at our peril.[6]

Are there areas in your life where you are attempting to live beyond your limits? How will you begin to practice "letting go and letting God"?

_____

_____

_____

_____

_____

Father, even though I've never seen limits as a good thing before,
I promise to try and live within the limits You ordained for me in this life.
In Christ's name, Amen.

Day
7

REFLECTION AND APPLICATION

Speak, Lord, for Your servant is listening today. Really, I am.
In Christ's name, Amen.

Today your assignment is to *listen* to God. Focus on being quiet in solitude and in expectation that you will hear from the Lover of your soul. Take a blank notebook or journal with you and write down what you hear God saying to you. (You can write down your prayers/thoughts to Him as well.) Follow the advice of this wise older Christian:

> Years ago I learned to read a chapter in the Bible daily and journal about what I read. Now I also ask, "Lord, what do You want to say to me today?" Then I listen quietly for the Spirit. . . . The more aware we are that God speaks personally, the more important it is to read the Bible regularly and to apply discernment to what we are hearing. Knowing how to confirm God's voice adds greater certainty to my own decision making. Before I learned to distinguish what He was saying, I was sometimes fearful. I'd weigh pros and cons, ask for godly advice, and seek understanding from Scripture—but I didn't always have confidence I

was making the right choice. I still take those steps. Now I also expect the Holy Spirit to speak into the process, to confirm or deter, and to give me an inner settledness when I am on the right path. Because He leads me in choices day by day, I know I can count on Him to lead me in big matters too.[7]

What are three steps you can take to carve out time in your life to listen to God's voice?

_____

_____

_____

_____

_____

_____

Help me, almighty God, not to ever be so preoccupied with myself and my little world that I don't take time to be still and know that You are God. In Christ's name, Amen.

Notes

1. Regina Franklin, *Who Calls Me Beautiful?* (Grand Rapids, MI: Discovery House Publishers, 2004), p. 43.
2. Peter Scazzero, *Emotionally Healthy Spirituality* (Nashville, TN: Thomas Nelson Publishers, 2006), pp. 53-54.
3. Ibid.
4. Robert Benson, *The Echo Within* (Colorado Springs, CO: WaterBrook, 2009), pp. 56-57.
5. Mandisa, quoted in Camerin Courtney, "TCW Talks to Mandisa," *Today's Christian Woman*, July/August 2009, p. 18.
6. Richard A. Swenson, *The Overload Syndrome* (Colorado Springs, CO: NavPress, 1998), p. 37.
7. Roc Bottomly, "A God Who Speaks," *Discipleship Journal*, January/February 2009, p. 52.

Group Prayer Requests

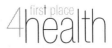

Today's Date: _____

Name	Request
Ann	Mr R. Grandaughter alter sound - give him a pase maker
Sure	God will pertect her.
Stacy	
Jody	Ken treamers

Results

_____

_____

_____

_____

_____

guard
the truth

SCRIPTURE MEMORY VERSE

Guard the good deposit that was entrusted to you—
guard it with the help of the Holy Spirit who lives in us.
2 TIMOTHY 1:14

God's purpose for you is that you walk with Him while here on earth and live with Him in heaven for all eternity. To that end, He has provided a way for you to do exactly that. In this week's memory verse, Paul encourages his friend Timothy and us to guard what has been entrusted to us: the truth of who God is, what He has done for us and how to live our lives in response to Him. Many people say they *believe* in God, but that doesn't necessarily mean they *trust* Him, *love* Him and *know* Him. Guarding the truth is more than just an intellectual practice. As our verse assures us, we have divine help to achieve this task of guarding the truth.

New Yorker Eric Metaxas, who speaks often to secular groups on Christian apologetics, writes the following in *Everything You Always Wanted to Know About God*:

So those who believe in God have to say that they trust in God, that they put their faith in Him, that they believe He is who the Bible says He is, and that He loves them more than they can ever imagine. If you know who God is, you will want to turn your will over to Him, because you trust Him with your life, you trust that His plans for you are far better than even the plans you've made for yourself. But if you don't really believe that God is the loving and wonderful God of the Bible who knows you intimately and loves you passionately, you'll never feel free to trust Him with your life.[1]

Day 1

KNOW TRUTH

Heavenly Father, help me today to know You better and to understand everything You've revealed about Yourself. In Christ's name, Amen.

Read Colossians 1:15-23. The Bible teaches that Jesus didn't merely have God-like abilities, but that He actually *was* God—Creator and Sustainer of the Universe. It is important to understand this foundational truth of Christ.

What two descriptions of Him are given in verse 15?

He is the _____

He is the _____

What did He create?

_____

_____

_____

_____

_____

Look up the word "supremacy" and write the definition here:

_____

_____

_____

_____

_____

As you read verse 19, write down your thoughts about Christ's identity and purpose.

_____

_____

_____

_____

_____

Verses 21-22 refer to Christ's work of reconciliation by taking the punishment for our sin on Himself so that we might live in newness of life. Write down what that might look like in your own life (see v. 21).

_____

_____

_____

_____

_____

Now, since Christ died for your sins, how does He want to present you to the world (see v. 22)?

_____

_____

_____

_____

_____

But what is the condition of your walking and abiding in that truth (see v. 23)?

_____

_____

_____

_____

_____

When you have doubts about Jesus or the "good deposit" He has made in you, what is usually happening in your life?

_____

_____

_____

_____

What is one action you will take when you are experiencing doubt? Will you call someone?

_____

_____

_____

_____

Forgive me, Father, for sometimes treating You as only one option for my life. Thank You for embodying Absolute Truth. In Christ's name, Amen.

Day 2 EMBRACE TRUTH

Gracious God, I'm ready to grow in my relationship to You through the Trinity—the Father, Son and Holy Spirit. In Christ's name, Amen.

Is Christianity for you a religion or a relationship? Without a relationship with Jesus Christ at the core, Christianity becomes just a religion of rules and rituals. Have you ever viewed your own spiritual life in that way? Are you ready for more?

Read Romans 10:9-13,17. How does verse 9 say we can move from religion to relationship?

If you _____

and if you _____

then you _____.

What do you think is the importance of these two steps?

Confessing with the mouth

_____

_____

_____

Believing with the heart

_____

_____

_____

According to verse 17, where did our faith come from?

_____

_____

_____

_____

How does that help you understand why studying the Word is so important in seeking God's purpose for your life?

_____

_____

_____

_____

In order to fully embrace Truth, each person must personally make a decision for faith in Christ. Perhaps you have done this before—recently or very long ago. The important thing is that you have done it at some time so that you have the assurance of Jesus Christ living inside you.

Gracious God, thank You that I can be assured that You are with me each day. When my life on earth is over, I will dwell with You in heaven for all eternity. In Christ's name, Amen.

ON GUARD!

Dear God, help me to stay awake and alert so that I don't get slack in my pursuit of You and Your purpose. In Christ's name, Amen.

In the first two days of this week, we have examined the gospel message and been given an opportunity to respond to Christ's invitation to make Him Lord of our lives. Living by this truth is a daily choice to follow what God lays out as His will through His Word.

Read Proverbs 7:1-3. What commands are given in these verses?

_____

_____

_____

What is one way you can "store up My commands within you"?

_____

_____

_____

Recall a time during the past nine weeks when one of your First Place 4 Health memory verses came to mind just when you needed it.

_____

_____

_____

What about a time when you were able to share the message of a verse with someone else?

_____

_____

_____

What do you think Proverbs 7:3 means?

_____

_____

_____

_____

Pastor Chuck Swindoll endorses Scripture memory and shares the following benefits: "I know of no other single practice in the Christian life more rewarding, practically speaking, than memorizing scripture. . . . No other single exercise pays greater spiritual dividends! Your prayer life will be strengthened. Your witnessing will be sharper and much more effective. Your counseling will be in demand. Your attitudes and outlook will begin to change. Your mind will become alert and observant. Your confidence and assurance will be enhanced. Your faith will be solidified."[2]

Read 2 Peter 3:17-18. One of the reasons we are admonished to guard the truth is that others seek to steal our joy or lead us astray through questioning, temptation and doubts. What does Peter advise we do?

_____

_____

_____

_____

In verse 18, we are encouraged to grow in two major areas of the Christian life. What are they, and what does each term mean?

Grow in _____

_____

_____

Grow in _____

_____

_____

As you grow in grace and knowledge, here are some practical suggestions for your new walk of faith:

1. Pray constantly. Prayer is simply talking to Jesus. Be sure to include praise, thanksgiving, confession of sins, requests for help and petitions for others.

2. Read your Bible. Be sure you put God's Word into your heart every day. If you don't know where to begin, start with the Gospel of John.

3. Worship with others. It's difficult to live out the Christian life alone. Meet with a church family where the Bible is taught and obeyed and Jesus Christ is Lord and Savior.

4. Witness to others. Tell your friends what Christ has done for you, remembering that people respond to actual stories of what God has done in our lives.

Father, You know these four practices are hard for me to keep up each day, but I know You will help me in my spiritual disciplines. Amen.

Day
4

GUIDANCE AND FREEDOM

Lord, I have so many questions and pray that You will show me the way to take in all my decision making today. In Christ's name, Amen.

Read John 16:13. When you are searching for truth, where do you usually turn?

_____

_____

_____

_____

What part does the Holy Spirit play in bearing the truth (see v. 13)?

_____

_____

_____

_____

In what area of your life do you most need guidance today?

_____

_____

_____

_____

Write a prayer, asking God to guide you into all truth for that area of your life:

_____

_____

_____

_____

_____

Read John 8:31-33. According to this passage, how do others know that we are followers of Christ (that is, "disciples")?

_____

_____

_____

_____

And what will be the result of our actions?

_____

_____

_____

_____

_____

Do you feel *free* right now, or is there something that has imprisoned you, holding you back from full freedom in Christ? From what/whom do you need to be freed?

_____

_____

_____

_____

Now, find a scriptural promise (it could be from this very Bible study in past weeks) that speaks of the *truth* that can free you. (If you need help, try searching for key words in a Bible concordance, such as "guilt," "regret," "idolatry," and so on.)

_____

_____

_____

_____

Today, pray that you can begin to embrace God's truth, which will truly set you free.

Gracious God, please grant me true freedom from You-know-what.
I'm ready to end this slavery. In Christ's name, Amen.

Day
5

FIRM FAITH

Almighty God, I want to be one of those folk who never falter in their faith,
so would You give me extra courage today? In Christ's name, Amen.

Read 1 Timothy 6:19-21. What is the "treasure" referred to in this passage?

_____

_____

_____

_____

What is the purpose behind laying up this treasure?

_____

_____

_____

Once again we read about "guarding what has been entrusted." Why do you think there is so much warning imagery here?

_____

_____

_____

What specifically are we advised to turn away from (see v. 20)?

_____

_____

_____

What does "godless chatter" look like in your life?

_____

_____

_____

Do you know some who have "wandered from the faith"? How and why do you think that happened?

_____

_____

_____

Paul ends with the blessing, "Grace be with you." You may be aware that your First Place 4 Health group leader is praying for you and others are as well. Are you praying for them? E. M. Bounds writes the following about prayer:

> True prayer that wins an answer must be backed up by a scriptural, vital, personal religion. They are the essentials of real Christian service in this life. Of these requirements the most important is that in serving, we serve. So in praying, we must talk with God. Truth and heart reality, these are the core, the substance, the sum, the heart of prayer. Prayer has no potential unless we pray with simplicity, sincerity and truth.

End by praying simply, sincerely and honestly for your fellow First Place 4 Health travelers. Use the space below or your journal to record some words of blessing you will say to one or two of them this week.

_____

_____

_____

_____

Thank You, Jesus, for sitting right beside me and listening to every concern and request in my prayers. In Christ's name, Amen.

Day 6

REFLECTION AND APPLICATION

Lord, help me to put one step in front of the other today and then to keep walking in the right direction with You by my side. In Christ's name, Amen.

The journey of faith is, someone once said, "a long obedience in the same direction." In other words, we must keep putting one foot in front of the other, obeying God by continuing on as we've been taught. The great news is that we have a Companion with us on this long walk: God the Father, His Son Jesus Christ and the Holy Spirit (the Trinity).

Don't you love taking walks with someone else? It seems to make the time pass more quickly—and learning to pace ourselves with another is always a great discipline. This is part of what we have been learning through First Place 4 Health: that we don't have to go it alone.

By now you know that First Place 4 Health is not a diet, because the first three letters in that word are D-I-E. Instead, we refer to our journey as the Live It Plan. The path we seek to walk is a balanced life where Christ is given first place. As a reminder, here are the four areas of balance:

1. Physical balance comes when you learn to enjoy eating healthy foods—not because you're trying to lose weight, but because the foods taste good and they make you feel good. Regular exercise is a vital key to physical balance because it improves your health while regulating daily stress.

2. Mental balance comes when you learn to change your thinking about God, yourself, relationships and health. Changing how you think changes who you are. Memorizing God's Word and using resources such as this Bible study help you develop new ways of thinking, not only about weight loss, but also about who you are as a person.

3. Emotional balance comes when you learn that no thing—including high-fat, high-sugar foods—can ever fill the empty place in your heart, because that space was made for God. He will heal as you face head-on your grief-causing behaviors.

4. Spiritual balance comes as you seek God ahead of all other desires. Spiritual disciplines, such as prayer, Bible Study and Scripture memory, help you achieve a life of spiritual balance, full of love, joy and peace.[3]

> *Father, when we live in true balance, we don't fall over as much.*
> *Show me if one of these four areas is weak and causing me to topple.*
> *Thank You, Lord. In Christ's name, Amen.*

REFLECTION AND APPLICATION

*Lord, help me to incorporate spiritual disciplines into my life so that I may
stay close to You and grow in godliness. In Christ's name, Amen.*

Read Psalm 25:4-6. Use this Scripture to offer a prayer of petition to God:

Show me _____

Teach me _____

Guide me _____

Teach me _____

My hope _____

Remember _____

Try to take an extra amount of time to be quiet before God today. Solitude and sanctuary are important aspects of our spiritual lives, yet are often neglected due to constant demands from others. Get in the habit of
scheduling time for Sabbath rest, preferably on a Sunday. As Dallas
Willard states:

> My central claim is that we can become like Christ by doing one
> thing—by following Him in the overall style of life He chose for
> Himself. If we have faith in Christ, we must believe that He knew
> how to live. We can, through faith and grace, become like Christ
> by practicing the types of activities He engaged in by arranging
> our whole lives around the activities He Himself practiced in or-
> der to remain constantly at home in the fellowship of His Father.
>
> What activities did Jesus practice? Such things as solitude
> and silence, prayer, simple and sacrificial living, intense study and
> meditation upon God's Word and God's ways, and service to oth-
> ers. Some of them will certainly be even more necessary to us than
> they were to Him, because of our greater or different need.
>
> So, if we wish to follow Christ—and to walk in the easy yoke
> with Him—we will have to accept His overall way of life as our

way of life totally. Then, and only then, we may reasonably expect to know by experience how easy is the yoke and how light the burden.[5]

What are three spiritual disciplines you will incorporate into your journey with God?

_____

_____

_____

_____

_____

_____

Almighty God, may I seek regular times for solitude and silence even though that goes against my nature. In Christ's name, Amen.

Notes

1   Eric Metaxas, *Everything You Always Wanted to Know About God* (Colorado Springs, CO: WaterBrook Press, 2005), p. 174.

2. Charles Swindoll, *Growing Strong in the Seasons of Life* (Portland OR: Multnomah Press, 1983), p. 78.

3. Adapted from Carole Lewis, *The Divine Diet* (Ventura, CA: Gospel Light Publishers, 2004) pp. 12-13.

4. Dallas Willard, *Spirit of the Disciplines: Understanding How God Changes Lives* (San Francisco, CA: Harper and Row, 1988), p. 8.

Group Prayer Requests

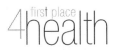

Today's Date: _____

Name	Request
Anon	preachers son Depression Sue & Betty
Tony	finances, Sara, her new Job.
Sue	her daughter, wants to hang on tight
Linda	Daughter in law her attitude
Joy	Show Joy what she needs to Ken work on
Stacy	Court date three days meadtation

Results

_____

_____

_____

_____

_____

declare personal victory

SCRIPTURE MEMORY VERSE
*But you are a chosen people, a royal priesthood, a holy nation,
a people belonging to God, that you may declare the praises
of him who called you out of darkness into his wonderful light.*
1 PETER 2:9

Let's look at all God has done over the past weeks as we have sought His purpose for our lives. Perhaps we haven't achieved all our goals or perhaps we have surpassed them, but we all have some personal victory to declare. In our memory verse, Peter points out four different sources of our identity. What are they?

1. You are a *Chosen people*
2. You are a *royal Priesthood*
3. You are a *holy nation*
4. You are a *people belonging to God.*

Have you ever thought of yourself in these terms? How does it make you feel as you consider these descriptions?

It makes me fell very Blessed, And very Close to God.

How do you think embracing our true identity as described in this verse should lead us to action?

We should wante to live the life he has given uses. Holy before him

Are you ready to declare personal victory? Why or why not?

Yes I am. I speak victory over my Children over today my life, Bills

SPEAK UP

Show me, Father, all the victories You have been working in my life so far.
In Christ's name, Amen.

Read 2 Corinthians 4:13-18. The word "therefore" in this Scripture passage is almost like an equal sign (=). Thus viewed, how would you fill in this equation (using verse 13)?

I _____ = I _____

We _____ = We _____

How do you feel about speaking of what God has done in your life?

_____

_____

_____

People can argue with our theology, but they can't dispute our testimony of what actually happened in our lives. That's why sharing true stories is so important. What does verse 15 say the intended outcome is from sharing your testimony?

_____

_____

_____

_____

_____

Are you ever tempted to "lose heart"? List what verse 16 says as:

Reason to *lose* heart: _____

Reason to *take* heart: _____

As you look back at these three months of Bible study, list your own:

Reasons to *lose* heart

_____

_____

_____

_____

Reasons to *take* heart

_____

_____

_____

_____

Now list your own "light and momentary troubles."

_____

_____

_____

_____

_____

According to verse 17, why are those troubles in your life?

_____

_____

_____

Perhaps you think you are not as far along the path of balanced health as you want to be. But remember: What you see is not all there is to reality! How is that elaborated on in verse 18?

_____

_____

_____

_____

Heavenly Father, truly there are things to share with others, and I'm so grateful that You will help me speak up with good news. In Christ's name, Amen.

Day 2

GOD'S INDWELLING

Thank You, Lord, for coming into my heart and living within me so that I might be able to do far more than I ever could have done alone. Amen.

Read Philippians 2:12-18. God's purpose is stated clearly in the first part of verse 16. Write it here:

_____

_____

_____

_____

In order to "hold out" or share the "word of life" better, we must have God living inside us. What great promise can we count on (see v. 13)?

_____

_____

_____

_____

What does God call us to continue to do (see vv. 12 and 14)?

_____

_____

_____

When you complain or argue with others—or even God—what is it usually about?

_____

_____

_____

_____

When you abstain from complaining and arguing, what godly qualities result in your life (see v. 15)?

_____

_____

_____

_____

If we are faithful to the God who is faithful to us, what two things should characterize our lives (see v. 18)?

1. _____

2. _____

What are several things for which you can rejoice?

_____

_____

_____

_____

Gracious Provider of all things, may I always have a thankful heart
for the many blessings You have sent my way. In Christ's name, Amen.

Day
3

SENT BY GOD

Lord, You have called me and You will send me and, by Your grace,
I will follow where You lead. In Christ's name, Amen.

By now you have probably grown comfortable with the folks in your
Bible study group and entered a certain level of familiarity and understanding. How great it would be if the fellowship and sharing could always continue! Perhaps they can, either with this group or in another
time and place. But growing and learning together is not all God has
purposed for His followers. Read Jeremiah 1:4-10. He also calls us to go
out into the world. How is this concept described in verse 5?

_____

_____

_____

_____

What is your usual response when you feel God is asking you to do a
hard thing?

_____

_____

_____

_____

Often, we feel inadequate about speaking of faith matters to others. When
Jeremiah protested that he was too young and inexperienced to do what
God commanded, what six things did God say in response (see vv. 7-9)?

Do not say _____

You must go _____

You must say _____

Do not be _____

I am _____

I will _____

God will put His words into your mouth! The following is a great exercise to help you prepare a short testimony of what God has done in your life. The prompts are designed to give you specific ideas for formulating your own testimony. After you complete each one, combine them in one testimony—remembering that short and simple are the best way to communicate. Practice sharing it, and then when the time comes, you'll be ready!

My life before following Christ . . .

_____

_____

_____

How God broke through to change me . . .

_____

_____

_____

My life today as a follower of Christ (include one or two important spiritual lessons and some encouragement) . . .

_____

_____

_____

In verse 10 of Jeremiah 1, God reveals His purpose for Jeremiah's life, which includes an appointment to do six things:

1. _____
2. _____
3. _____
4. _____
5. _____
6. _____

Is there one of these that might apply to your life's purpose, too? Explain.

_____

_____

_____

_____

Thanks, God, for the story You have woven throughout my life. Please help me share it often, with humility and purpose. In Christ's name, Amen.

Day
4

WHAT GOD CAN DO

You do so much, Heavenly Father, and we so rarely praise You for such amazing things. Today I choose to praise and thank You. Amen.

Read Psalm 146:1-10. As we continue to examine ways to declare personal victory in our lives, it's important to give all glory to God. Psalm 146 begins with a litany of praise to Jehovah-Jirah—the Lord who provides. Begin today with your own litany of praise. Use Psalm 146 as inspiration.

_____

_____

_____

_____

In verses 3-4, we are warned against what? Explain.

_____

_____

_____

_____

What are the reasons given in verses 5-6 for our being blessed by God?

_____

_____

_____

_____

There is mention of at least 11 instances of God's faithfulness in verses 7-10. List them here. The Lord:

1. _____
2. _____
3. _____
4. _____
5. _____
6. _____
7. _____
8. _____
9. _____
10. _____
11. _____

As you look at this list, identify which actions God has done or continues to do for you today, and thank Him for them.

> *Faithful One, thank You for never giving up on me—especially in these past months as I am seeking to live a healthier life on all levels. Amen.*

USED BY GOD   Day 5

> *Lord, sometimes pouring myself out for others gets tiring, but I'm so grateful that You continue to refresh me anew each day. In Christ's name, Amen.*

Read Isaiah 58:9-12. This powerful passage of Scripture clearly shows how God's people are to act in partnership with Him. He longs to use us but we must be willing and prepared to be used by God. What are the promises in the first part of verse 9?

You will _____ and the Lord will _____

You will _____ and the Lord will say _____

Later, in verses 9-10 there are more instructions for cause and effect:

If you _____ ,
with the _____ ,
and if you _____
and _____ ,
then _____ ,
and _____ .

Often in our lives we feel spent, used up and totally exhausted from expending energy and resources on things that have no real value. In God's economy, we are actually energized when we pour out our lives. Verse 11 gives five amazing ways God does this.

The Lord will _____
The Lord will _____
The Lord will _____
The Lord will make you _____
The Lord will make you _____

Water images imply a sense of refreshment and reinvigoration. Which of the above five speaks most to your heart today and why?

_____
_____
_____
_____

Finally, God gives us a big task (see v. 12). God's people are to:

Rebuild _____
Raise up _____
Be called _____
Be called _____

Gracious God, I am humbled that You want to use me to accomplish great things for Your kingdom. I am Yours and I am willing. Amen.

REFLECTION AND APPLICATION

Help me, precious Lord, to keep going even when I feel disillusioned or discouraged, knowing that You are not finished with me yet. Amen.

Now that we have looked at all God has done and all we have done, the question is, *Can we keep on going—step by step—living a balanced life in God's will and God's way?* The answer can be a resounding yes! By the grace of God, we can! In Philippians 1:6, Paul states that the source of his confidence is that "He who began a good work in [us] will carry it on to completion until the day of Christ Jesus." Our part in the walk of faith is to keep walking. Look up the definition of "perseverance" and write it here:

_____

_____

_____

_____

_____

Are you ever worried that you won't be able to continue the commitments and growth you have experienced spiritually, physically, mentally and emotionally when your 12 weeks in *God's Purpose for You* is over? If so, what do you believe is the source of that concern?

_____

_____

_____

_____

Isaiah 50:7 reminds us that the Sovereign Lord helps us: "I will not be _____!" However, he says he must do something (see v. 7b). What is that?

_____

_____

_____

_____

What do you think that means?

_____

_____

_____

_____

Shame is a powerful weapon used by the enemy of our souls to destroy our will and dismantle our fortitude. Do not give in to shame!

Thank You, Lord, for delivering me from shame and reminding me that I do not have to live there anymore! In Christ's name, Amen.

Day 7

REFLECTION AND APPLICATION

May my life be one of victory and power, as You fill me, Lord, to overflowing with Yours. In Christ's name, Amen.

This week has been all about victory. Think of each of the past six days and jot down one idea from each study that you'd like to remember.

Day 1: "Speak Up"

_____

_____

_____

Day 2: "God's Indwelling"

_____

_____

_____

Day 3: "Sent by God"

_____

_____

_____

Day 4: "What God Can Do"

_____

_____

_____

Day 5: "Used by God"

_____

_____

_____

Day 6: "Perseverance"

_____

_____

_____

Write down some personal victories you have experienced as you have studied *God's Purpose for You:*

_____

_____

_____

_____

_____

_____

_____

This is not the end, but merely the close of one leg of your ongoing journey. Your story is not over yet, and God has so much more ahead for His children. May you be empowered to live victoriously and declare what God has done for you so that others might be encouraged in their own pursuits of a balanced life!

> *Almighty God, reveal Your purpose for every area of my life and I will be Yours forever, an obedient and grateful servant. In Christ's name, Amen.*

Group Prayer Requests

first place
4health

Today's Date: _____

Name	Request
Joy	Stacy health Defets her
Linda	
Sue	Georgie Ann Demincha. shes pray for her
Ann	put her trust in the Lord
Joy	Ken, God will bring him out of his discourged

Results

_____

_____

_____

_____

_____

time to
celebrate!

To help shape your brief victory celebration testimony, work through the following questions in your prayer journal:

Day One: List some of the benefits you have gained by allowing the Lord to transform your life through this 12-week First Place 4 Health session. Be sure to list benefits you have received in the physical, mental, emotional and spiritual realms of your being.

Day Two: In what ways have you most significantly changed *mentally*? Have you seen a shift in the ways you think about yourself, food, your relationships or God? How has Scripture memory been a part of these shifts?

Day Three: In what ways have you most significantly changed *emotionally*? Have you begun to identify how your feelings influence your relationship to food and exercise? What are you doing to stay aware of your emotions, both positive and negative?

Day Four: In what ways have you most significantly changed *spiritually*? How has your relationship with God deepened? How has drawing closer to Him made a difference in the other three areas of your life?

Day Five: In what ways have you most significantly changed *physically*? Have you met or exceeded your weight/measurement goals? How has your health improved the past 12 weeks?

Day Six: Was there one person in your First Place 4 Health group who was particularly encouraging to you? How did their kindness make a difference in your First Place 4 Health journey?

Day Seven: Summarize the previous six questions into a one-page testimony, or "faith story," to share at your group's victory celebration.

May our gracious Lord bless and keep you as you continue to keep Him first in all things!

God's Purpose for You
leader discussion guide

For in-depth information, guidance and helpful tips about leading a successful First Place 4 Health group, study the *First Place 4 Health Leader's Guide*. In it, you will find valuable answers to most of your questions, as well as personal insights from many First Place 4 Health group leaders.

For the group meetings in this session, be sure to read and consider each week's discussion topics several days before the meeting—some questions and activities require supplies and/or planning to complete. Also, if you are leading a large group, plan to break into smaller groups for discussion and then come together as a large group to share your answers and responses. Make sure to appoint a capable leader for each small group so that discussions stay focused and on track (and be sure each group records their answers!).

week one: welcome to *God's purpose for you*

During this first week, welcome the members to your group, provide a brief overview of the First Place 4 Health program, explain what is expected of the participants at each of the weekly meetings, and collect the Member Surveys. (See the *First Place 4 Health Leader's Guide* for a detailed outline of how to conduct the first week's meeting.)

week two: respond wholeheartedly

Ask the group members to pinpoint ways their lives might have been "running wild" before they decided to join First Place 4 Health. What sorts of restraint had they cast off? Discuss whether or not boundaries and laws are a good thing.

During this week's study, members looked up the word "revelation." Discuss the definition and how it applies to what God reveals to us as His will and His way. Why don't more people understand this concept?

Have someone read Psalm 73:21-28 and then discuss phrases that members of the group might feel expresses where they are or have been.

Go over each of the four health areas—physical, mental, spiritual and emotional—and have members share what they believe God's way is for us in each of those areas. (It's especially good if they have a Scripture to back up what they are saying.)

Have the group share "triggers" that become obstacles for obedience as they seek to follow this new lifestyle of balanced health. Write the answers on a board, go through the list of the group's "triggers," and then put a plan of action next to it that they could take when tempted.

Recite together this week's memory verse and discuss why First Place 4 Health emphasizes Scripture memory. Read the letter found on Day 5 from the new participant who is seeking to follow the program. Ask the group if they have ever "dabbled" before and where that got them.

Talk about the commitment, based on Psalm 119:111-112, that the members had an opportunity to sign on Day 5. What will it take for them to stay wholehearted their whole lives?

Ask if anyone wants to share his or her own story of God's revelation? How did God finally get that person's attention and spur him or her on to pursuing a healthier life?

week three: desire real change

Ask participants to discuss some of the hardest times of change they have encountered in their lives so far and how they handled those changes. Did it make a difference if it was change they chose or change that just happened to them?

Ask members if they found it uncomfortable or awkward to identify their deepest desires. Was it hard to write them down? Why?

Have someone read the story of the man at the pool of Bethesda in John 5:1-9. What are some of the group's reactions to that story?

Does anyone believe that Jesus is asking him or her, "Do you want to get well?" If so, what is that person's answer?

Ask for a volunteer to explain the metamorphosis of a caterpillar to a butterfly. Then point out that change of that kind is what we called "transformation." A caterpillar doesn't become a faster caterpillar, but a totally new creature—one that can soar. Paul uses this same root word (*metamorphoo*) to describe what God wants to do in transforming us—changing from the inside out. Ask the group to dream about the totally new creature they could become with this kind of transformation. Have them draw a picture that gives hints of that result. (Note: the drawing doesn't have to be of their new body; it could be a pair of running shoes or a new hairdo or a symbol of a trip or anything that might reflect the goal they hope to achieve.)

Ask participants if they have appropriated the Holy Spirit's power that is available for every follower of Christ. Have them try to identify the difference that might occur in various areas of their lives by comparing "in our own power" versus "through God's power of the Holy Spirit."

Discuss where they have gone to seek life rather than to God. Do they have something else to replace that now that they've been learning about living a balanced life? Ask for examples.

Ask members to pair up as partners (or use their prayer partners if they already have paired up for that) and have each person identify one change he or she hopes to see by the end of this 12-week session. Ask the pairs to commit to praying daily about that change in their partner.

Close with a reading of Jeremiah 29:11 and a prayer.

week four: love God totally

Share ways each of us can love God by going daily into each of the "four rooms of our house" (see Day 2)—body, soul, mind and spirit.

On Day 3, members read that we love God by keeping His commands. Discuss what are we saying to God when we don't keep His commands. Which of God's commands are especially hard for the members to keep?

Ask if anyone cares to share briefly (no names, please) his or her own experience with a "frenemy." What can such encounters teach us about how our actions speak volumes with regard to our love for God?

Ask each member to share one thing God has done for him or her out of His great love. Next, ask the group as a whole when the last time they shared with someone else how God has loved them. Challenge them to seek an opportunity to do so this week.

Read 1 John 4:17-21 and ask who might want to share some of the fears they wrote about on Day 6.

Discuss why is it important that those who love God also love others.

Have a volunteer read the definitions of "omniscient," "omnipotent" and "omnipresent" from Day 7. Ask the group to share which of these attributes they most appreciate or need from God this week.

End your session by asking everyone to close his or her eyes while one person reads aloud the love letter from God on Day 7.

week five: stand strong

Go around the group and ask the group to share aloud one of the strongholds they identified on Day 1. Mention that they are allowed to say "pass" if they prefer not to share.

Have a volunteer read Ephesians 6:10-18, and then go over the table everyone completed on Day 1, emphasizing what spiritual armor does for us.

Ask for volunteers to share how they felt on Day 2 about identifying Satan as an enemy, villain and foe.

Review the five ways God comes to us in strength (see the list on Day 3). Have participants discuss which particular ones speak to them, and why.

Ask for a volunteer to share why King David talked so much about God protecting and rescuing him. Refer to lists on Day 4 and point out ways that God did this. Next, go over your own lists from Day 4 and share similarly what God is doing to keep you strong.

On Day 6, members were asked if there is anything they need to lay aside in order to pursue their relationship with God. What did some of the members identify?

Soldiers of the Roman Empire became lazy and undisciplined, until eventually they were unable to sustain victorious strength (see Day 7). Ask members what they are doing daily to prepare so that they will prevail as battles arise.

week six: receive divine power

Often we complain about how hard it is to lead a godly life, yet our memory verse this week says we have everything we need to do just that. Discuss some of the reasons why we still struggle.

Share from your notes on Days 1 and 2 how you can use the Spirit's power in your own life. Name some instances when relying on willpower alone caused you to fail at balanced healthy living.

Ask volunteers to give examples from Day 3 of choices they made directed by their sinful nature. Contrast those choices with choices they could have made instead—choices directed by the Spirit.

Discuss why the Holy Spirit's identity as "Counselor" is appealing or not.

Have a group discussion concerning their various struggles and accomplishments in the exercise arena during first six weeks.

Day 5 emphasized that true transformation must begin in our hearts and minds. Ask participants what hang-ups they have in those areas. Did Regina's story strike a chord in anyone?

When we are overstressed and agitated, we need to remind ourselves to breathe. Discuss why stopping to take a long breath is a step toward calm and serenity.

Go around the group and share specific distractions you each have. Then have someone read aloud the quote by Fil Anderson on Day 7.

Challenge each person to write down a time this coming week when they will seek God through solitude and silence.

week seven: look inward

Ask if anyone is willing to share how he or she turned to food (or any other substance/habit) to meet needs that only God can meet.

On Day 1, we were encouraged to ask God to bring into the light some things about us we had pushed deep into dark corners of our lives. Ask if anyone would be willing to share this process.

Have a volunteer read Ephesians 2:1-10, and ask the members which verse in that section spoke loudest to them, and why.

Ask members it they agree with the statement that if we truly embraced the meaning of Ephesians 2:8-9, our lives would be changed forever. Why or why not? What do they now believe about God's grace in their lives?

Discuss some of the consequences those in the group experienced before beginning their journey to balanced health.

Ask if anyone in the group can relate to Mandisa's story on Day 2 of how she responded when she was humiliated on *American Idol*. What was the "takeaway" for them?

It's a great blessing that we can go directly to God at all times in all places. As you review Day 5, share some ways with the group that they can make "spiritual deposits" in God's presence.

Ask members to share how definitions of beauty influenced them while growing up, for better or for worse.

Ask participants to think of someone whose inner beauty attracts him or her to them (see Day 6). What are those characteristics displayed, and how can each of us get them, too?

Have a volunteer read the biblical characters' quote on Day 7, and then ask the group to share the dream they each wrote down. Close with prayer for each person, their dream and God's purpose to be fulfilled in His way and timing.

week eight: overcome obstacles

How do the members identify with Paul's struggles of doing what he does not want to do and not doing what he knows he should do (see Day 1)?

Ask participants to describe the last time their own version of "Flesh Woman" or "Flesh Man" showed up and took over. What were the results?

Have the group share the particulars about a time when someone comforted them. What did they learn that will help them comfort someone else in the future?

Ask for volunteers in your group who either were adopted or have adopted a child to share their experience briefly. What do you think God wants to communicate to us through the adoption analogy we studied on Day 3?

Paul listed many of the obstacles that were powerful but still helpless to put a wedge between him and God (see Day 4). Ask members what encouragement this gives them. What obstacles are they up against on their journey to balanced health?

On Day 5, prayer is mentioned as a powerful weapon for those hoping to overcome the world. An example of prayer is given. Ask members to share other helpful prayers or places where they find prayers to sustain them.

Go around the circle and ask each person to share how he or she is "new" since beginning this study.

Close in prayer, suggesting that each person surrender to God any part of his or her life that he or she has been holding back and asking God to fill each person. Use the prayer from Day 7, "God, this day is for You."

week nine: listen to God's voice

Have group members share about the pros and cons of having a GPS system and how that relates to responding to God's voice.

Day 1 presents a sort of bad news/good news story of God and the Israelites. Ask members how they would describe it and what important points they are to take to heart from it.

Have members share a time when God shouted at them through a "megaphone of pain" (Day 2), and their eventual response.

Ask the group what negative messages from their past are still replayed occasionally in their minds. When they choose to believe those messages, what happens?

On Day 3, participants were asked to check off three positive statements they wanted to embrace this week. Go around and have each person share one each.

Have a volunteer read the quote about overload from Dr. Richard Swenson (see Day 6), and then ask people to share their current struggles and victories in this area.

Ask for volunteers to share the results of their time in solitude and silence (see Day 7) and how it impacted them. Take time to have everyone in the group jot down a note, planning a time for solitude and silence in the week ahead.

week ten: guard the truth

Ask participants if there was ever a time when they said they believed in God, but they realize now that at that time they didn't actually trust, love or know Him. What did they learn about Christ on Day 1's study of Scripture? Do they believe it's true?

If we are to guard the truth, we must first know the truth. Share some of your experiences so far with both the pitfalls and possibilities of Scripture memory (see Day 3).

Discuss why each of the four spiritual disciplines listed on Day 3 are important in the life of a growing Christian.

Discuss what each of us needs to do to experience true freedom from that which may still have us "in chains."

Have group members share ways they have learned to "walk in truth" in each of the four areas of health—physical, mental, spiritual and emotional.

On Day 7, participants were asked to "become like Christ by practicing the types of activities He engaged in." Can they think of an instance in which they have done this?

week eleven: declare personal victory

Ask the group which of the four sources of identity in this week's memory verse they feel the most comfortable with, and why.

Ask how people feel about the concept in Jeremiah 1 (see Day 3) of being sent by God to speak to others of spiritual things.

On Day 4, participants wrote out their own litany of praise to God for all that He has done for them in their lives. Go around the circle today and have each person fill in the following sentence: "Today, I praise God for _____."

Read Isaiah 58:9-12 and ask members to share how God has actually energized and refreshed them when they have served others.

Ask participants if they have both *confidence* and *perseverance,* and how they know.

Discuss how shame can be destructive in our lives. What can be done about this?

Go around the group and have each person pinpoint one thing they now believe is God's purpose for them. Close in a prayer of thanksgiving and commitment.

week twelve: time to celebrate!

Even though most of your meeting this week will be a victory celebration, take some time at the beginning of the meeting to talk about how much God loves each person in the group and how each of us is called to love our brothers and sisters in Christ. (See "Planning a Victory Celebration" in the *First Place 4 Health Leader's Guide* for ideas about throwing a successful celebration for your group.)

For the rest of the study time, allow each member to tell his or her *God's Purpose for You* story. Give members an equal opportunity to share the goals they set for themselves at the beginning of the session and talk about the challenges and good things God has done for them throughout the process. Don't allow the more talkative group members to monopolize all the time. Even the quiet members need an opportunity to share their stories and successes! Even those who have not met their goals have still been part of the journey, so allow them to share and talk about why they did not succeed.

Making a commitment to continue in First Place 4 Health is an important part of victory. Be sure to talk about your group's future plans, and make each person feel welcome to continue to journey with you.

First Place 4 Health menu plans

Each menu plan is based on approximately 1,400 to 1,500 calories per day. All recipe and menu exchanges were determined using the Master-Cook software, a program that accesses a database containing more than 6,000 food items prepared using the United States Department of Agriculture (USDA) publications and information from food manufacturers. As with any nutritional program, MasterCook calculates the nutritional values of the recipes based on ingredients. Nutrition may vary due to how the food is prepared, where the food comes from, soil content, season, ripeness, processing and method of preparation. For these reasons, please use the recipes and menu plans as approximate guides. Consult a physician and/or a registered dietitian before starting a weight-loss program.

For those who need more calories, add the following to the 1,400-calorie plan:

- 1,800 calories: 2 ounce equivalent of meat, 3 ounce equivalent of bread, $^1/_2$ cup vegetable serving, 1 tsp. fat

- 2,000 calories: 2 ounce equivalent of meat, 4 ounce equivalent of bread, $^1/_2$ cup vegetable serving, 3 tsp. fat

- 2,200 calories: 2 ounce equivalent of meat, 5 ounce equivalent of bread, $^1/_2$ cup vegetable serving, $^1/_2$ cup fruit serving, 5 tsp. fat

- 2,400 calories: 2 ounce equivalent of meat, 6 ounce equivalent of bread, 1 cup vegetable serving, $^1/_2$ cup fruit serving, 6 tsp. fat

First Week Grocery List

Produce
- [ ] alfalfa sprouts
- [ ] apples
- [ ] baby spinach
- [ ] baby spring mix (1 bag)
- [ ] bananas
- [ ] Bartlett pears
- [ ] broccoli
- [ ] butternut squash
- [ ] celery
- [ ] cucumber
- [ ] garlic
- [ ] ginger
- [ ] grapes
- [ ] green onions
- [ ] lettuce
- [ ] limes
- [ ] mango
- [ ] mixed berries
- [ ] mushrooms
- [ ] onions
- [ ] orange
- [ ] pineapple
- [ ] potatoes
- [ ] radishes
- [ ] red onion
- [ ] red potatoes
- [ ] romaine lettuce
- [ ] snow peas
- [ ] spinach
- [ ] sugar snap peas
- [ ] tangerine
- [ ] tomatoes
- [ ] watercress leaves
- [ ] watermelon

Baking Products
- [ ] bacon bits, imitation
- [ ] baking powder
- [ ] basil leaves
- [ ] blue cheese dressing
- [ ] canola oil
- [ ] chili garlic sauce
- [ ] chowchow
- [ ] cinnamon
- [ ] crushed red pepper
- [ ] dark sesame oil
- [ ] dried cranberries
- [ ] dried wild mushroom blend
- [ ] dry mustard
- [ ] flour
- [ ] ginger, bottled ground fresh
- [ ] honey
- [ ] ketchup
- [ ] lemon juice
- [ ] mirin
- [ ] nonstick cooking spray
- [ ] olive oil
- [ ] peach jam
- [ ] pepper, freshly ground black
- [ ] rice vinegar
- [ ] rosemary
- [ ] sage leaves
- [ ] salad dressing, light
- [ ] salad dressing, sweet and sour
- [ ] salt
- [ ] soy sauce, low-sodium
- [ ] sugar
- [ ] Sweet 'n Low®
- [ ] sweet pickle relish
- [ ] syrup, low-sugar

❏ thyme sprigs
❏ Tony Cachere Original Creole Seasoning®
❏ vanilla
❏ vegetable oil
❏ walnuts

Breads and Cereals
❏ baked chips
❏ bran muffin, fat-free
❏ bread, cinnamon-raisin
❏ bread, whole-wheat
❏ breadsticks
❏ buckwheat noodles
❏ cornmeal
❏ dinner rolls
❏ hamburger buns, whole-wheat
❏ Italian bread, Chicago-style
❏ oats, raw and uncooked
❏ penne pasta, whole-grain
❏ puffed-wheat cereal
❏ tortilla wraps, spinach or sun-dried tomato
❏ Wheat Chex®
❏ wide noodles

Canned Foods
❏ chicken broth, less-sodium
❏ Mandarin oranges
❏ peach slices, no sugar added

❏ 8-oz. pineapple chunks with juice (2 cans)

Dairy Products
❏ cream cheese, light
❏ eggs
❏ egg substitute
❏ margarine, reduced-calorie
❏ mayonnaise, light
❏ milk, nonfat
❏ milk, skim
❏ Muenster cheese
❏ orange juice
❏ Parmesan cheese
❏ yogurt, plain lowfat
❏ yogurt, plain nonfat

Frozen Foods
❏ frozen waffles, lowfat
❏ honey-glazed carrots
❏ Lean Cuisine Dinnertime Selects
❏ pizza crust

Meat and Poultry
❏ $1^1/_2$ lbs. beef
❏ chicken breasts
❏ 8 oz. deli ham
❏ 1 lb. ground sirloin
❏ 1 lb. sea scallops, large
❏ smoked turkey
❏ $1^1/_4$ lbs. tilapia

First Week Meals and Recipes

·

DAY 1

....

Breakfast

Apple Flapjacks

$3/4$ cup sifted flour
$1/2$ tsp. baking powder
$1/4$ tsp. cinnamon
$1^1/2$ tsp. vegetable oil
$1^1/2$ tsp. sugar

$1/4$ cup egg substitute
1 cup apple, finely chopped
$1/2$ cup skim milk
nonstick cooking spray

Sift flour with baking powder and cinnamon. Mix oil, sugar, egg substitute and apple. Combine wet and dry ingredients, gradually adding in milk. Spray a nonstick griddle with vegetable spray. Bake flapjacks on griddle as for pancakes. Sprinkle with brown sugar substitute if desired. Serves 4.

Nutritional Information: 202 calories; 5g fat (22.2% calories from fat); 7g protein; 33g carbohydrate; 2g dietary fiber; 1mg cholesterol; 143mg sodium.

....

Lunch

Chicken Salad Sandwiches

1 cup chopped cooked chicken breast
$1/3$ cup chopped cored apple,
   chopped seeded cucumber, or
   finely chopped celery
1 hard-cooked egg, peeled and
   chopped

2 tbsp. plain lowfat yogurt
2 tbsp. light mayonnaise or salad
   dressing
salt and black pepper
8 slices whole-wheat bread
4 lettuce leaves

In a medium bowl, stir together chicken, apple and egg. Add yogurt and mayonnaise and stir to combine. Season to taste with salt and pepper. Serve immediately or cover and chill up to 4 hours. Spread chicken mixture on half of the bread slices. Top with lettuce leaves and remaining bread slices. Cut away crusts if desired. Cut each sandwich into four triangles or squares. Serve with 1 ounce baked chips and 1 cup mixed berries.

Nutritional Information: 393 calories; 8g fat (20% calories from fat); 23g protein; 57g carbohydrate; 9g dietary fiber; 86mg cholesterol; 680mg sodium.

Dinner

Scallops with Soba Noodles with Steamed Peas Vinaigrette

3 tbsp. low-sodium soy sauce
1 tbsp. fresh orange juice
1 tbsp. rice vinegar
1 tbsp. honey
$1/2$ tsp. bottled ground fresh ginger
$1/4$ tsp. chili garlic sauce

1 tbsp. dark sesame oil, divided
1 lb. large sea scallops
4 cups hot cooked soba (about 6 oz. uncooked buckwheat noodles)
$1/8$ teaspoon salt
$1/4$ cup thinly sliced green onions

Combine soy sauce, orange juice, vinegar, honey, ginger, garlic sauce and 1 teaspoon oil in a shallow baking dish. Add scallops to the dish in a single layer. Marinate for 4 minutes on each side. Heat the remaining 2 teaspoons oil in a large skillet over medium-high heat. Remove scallops from dish, reserving marinade. Add scallops to pan and sauté for 1 minute on each side or until almost done. Remove scallops from the pan and keep warm. Place remaining marinade in pan and bring to a boil. Return scallops to pan and cook 1 minute. Toss noodles with salt and green onions. Place 1 cup noodle mixture on each of 4 plates. Top each serving with about 3 scallops and drizzle with 1 tablespoon sauce. Serve with *Steamed Peas Vinaigrette*. Serves 4.

Steamed Peas Vinaigrette

Steam 1 cup snow peas and 1 cup trimmed sugar snap peas, covered, 3 minutes or until crisp-tender. Combine with $1/3$ cup thinly sliced radishes. Combine 1 tablespoon rice vinegar, 1 tablespoon soy sauce, 2 teaspoons canola oil, $11/2$ teaspoons mirin, $1/4$ teaspoon black pepper, and $1/8$ teaspoon kosher salt; stir with a whisk. Pour over peas mixture and toss.

Nutritional Information: 315 calories; 4.5g fat (13% calories from fat); 28g protein; 42.7g carbohydrate; 1.9g dietary fiber; 37mg cholesterol; 653mg sodium.

DAY 2

Breakfast

Cran-Apple Oatmeal

2 cups skim milk
$1/3$ cup dried cranberries

$1/2$ tsp. ground cinnamon
$1/4$ tsp. salt

1 cup oats, rolled (raw) and uncooked   1 chopped apple
2 packets Sweet 'n Low® sweetener or $^1/_2$ tsp. vanilla
   1 tsp. sugar

Combine milk, cranberries, cinnamon and salt in a medium saucepan. Bring to a boil over medium heat, stirring occasionally. Add oats and apple. Simmer uncovered for 5 to 6 minutes for old-fashioned oats or 1 to 2 minutes for quick oats, stirring occasionally until most of liquid has been absorbed. Remove from heat. Stir in sweetener/sugar and vanilla. Serves 2.

Nutritional Information: 287 calories; 3g fat (10% calories from fat); 15g protein; 50g carbohydrate; 6g dietary fiber; 4mg cholesterol; 398mg sodium.

....

Lunch
Wendy's Chili® (8 oz.) $^1/_2$ packet of light dressing
side salad

Nutritional Information: 256 calories; 6g fat (25.2% calories from fat); 17g protein; 24g carbohydrate; 9g dietary fiber; 40mg cholesterol; 858mg sodium.

....

Dinner

Steak Salad Wraps
1$^1/_2$ lb. seasoned beef for fajitas   1 bag baby spring mix
$^1/_2$ cup blue cheese dressing   8 spinach or sun-dried tomato
2 tomatoes, chopped   tortilla wraps
1 small red onion, thinly sliced   nonstick cooking spray

On the grill: Spray the grill rack with nonstick cooking spray. Prepare charcoal or gas grill for cooking. Place fajitas on the grill rack. Cook each side for 8 to 10 minutes or until fully cooked. Cut meat across the grain into $^1/_2$-inch strips. In the skillet: Cut meat across the grain into $^1/_2$-inch strips. Heat skillet for three minutes over high heat. Spray a pan with nonstick cooking. Cook beef, stirring every 2 to 3 minutes until meat is fully cooked. Place cooked fajita meat on one end of large serving platter. Arrange blue cheese dressing, tomatoes, onion, spring mix, and spinach or sun-dried-tomato tortilla wraps on the other end of the platter. Let everyone combine his or her own wrap. Serve with 1 cup *Mixed Fruit Salad*. Serves 8.

Mixed Fruit Salad

2 bananas, sliced
(2) 8-oz. cans of pineapple chunks
with juice

2 apples, diced
2 cups grapes

Combine all and serve. (Note: pineapple juice keeps fruit salad fresh for three days.)

Nutritional Information: 475 calories; 19g fat (35.8% calories from fat); 19g protein; 57g carbohydrate; 7g dietary fiber; 52mg cholesterol; 568mg sodium.

DAY 3

Breakfast

2 lowfat frozen waffles, heated
1 tsp. reduced-calorie margarine
1 tbsp. low-sugar syrup

$1/2$ small mango
1 cup nonfat milk

Nutritional Information: 345 calories; 8g fat (20.6% calories from fat); 13g protein; 57g carbohydrate; 4g dietary fiber; 27mg cholesterol; 698mg sodium.

Lunch

Grilled Chicken and Pineapple Sandwiches

4 (6-oz.) skinless, boneless chicken
breast halves
$1/2$ tsp. salt
$1/4$ tsp. freshly ground black pepper
$1/4$ cup fresh lime juice (about 2
limes)

4 ($1/2$-inch-thick) slices fresh pineapple
4 ($11/2$-oz.) whole-wheat hamburger
buns, toasted
light mayonnaise (optional)
4 large basil leaves
nonstick cooking spray

Prepare grill. Sprinkle chicken evenly with salt and pepper. Place chicken on grill rack coated with nonstick cooking spray. Grill 5 to 6 minutes on each side or until done, brushing occasionally with lime juice. Grill pineapple 2 to 3 minutes on each side or until browned. Spread mayonnaise on bottom halves of buns, if desired. Top each with 1 chicken breast half, 1 pineapple slice, 1 basil leaf, and 1 bun top. Serve with 1 oz. baked chips. Serves 4.

Nutritional Information: 444 calories; 5g fat (12.8% calories from fat); 47.4g protein; 52.5g carbohydrate; 6.1g dietary fiber; 99mg cholesterol; 770mg sodium.

Dinner

Quick Meat Loaf

$1/_3$ cup chopped green onions
3 tbsp. dry breadcrumbs
2 tsp. minced garlic
$1/_2$ tsp. salt
$1/_2$ tsp. dry mustard
$1/_4$ tsp. freshly ground black pepper

$1/_4$ tsp. crushed red pepper
1 lb. ground sirloin
1 large egg, lightly beaten
6 tbsp. ketchup, divided
nonstick cooking spray

Preheat oven to 400° F. Combine ingredients in a large bowl and add $1/_4$ cup ketchup. Mix beef mixture with hands just until combined. Shape beef mixture into a 9" x 4" loaf on a broiler pan coated with nonstick cooking spray. Bake at 400° F for 20 minutes. Brush top of meat loaf with remaining 2 tablespoons ketchup. Bake 7 additional minutes or until done. Slice loaf into 8 equal pieces. Serve with 1 cup roasted red potatoes, 1 cup steamed broccoli with 1 tsp. light margarine and 1 dinner roll. Serves 4.

Nutritional Information: 500 calories; 15.1g fat (42.8% calories from fat); 33.6g protein; 57.8g carbohydrate; 6.7g dietary fiber; 127mg cholesterol; 856mg sodium.

DAY 4

Breakfast

Pear-Walnut Sandwiches

$1/_2$ cup (4 oz.) tub-style light cream cheese
8 (1.1-oz.) slices cinnamon-raisin bread, toasted
1 cup alfalfa sprouts

2 tbsp. finely chopped walnuts, toasted
2 Bartlett pears, cored and thinly sliced

Spread 1 tablespoon of cream cheese evenly over each of 8 bread slices. Sprinkle $1/_2$ tablespoon of walnuts evenly over each of 4 bread slices. Top each evenly with pear slices, sprouts, and 1 bread slice. Cut each sandwich in half diagonally. Serve with 1 cup nonfat milk. Serves 4.

Nutritional Information: 421 calories; 11g fat (22.8% calories from fat); 16.7g protein; 64.2g carbohydrate; 5.2g dietary fiber; 19mg cholesterol; 489mg sodium.

Lunch

Sliced Egg Salad

2 slices whole-wheat bread
1/4 cup watercress leaves or romaine
   lettuce

1 hard-boiled egg, sliced
2 tomato slices
2 tsp. light mayonnaise

Serve with 1/2 cup each carrot and celery sticks and a 3″ x 2″ wedge of watermelon. Serves 1.

Nutritional Information: 449 calories; 12g fat (22.8% calories from fat); 17g protein; 75g carbohydrate; 12g dietary fiber; 216mg cholesterol; 515mg sodium.

Dinner

Lean Cuisine Dinnertime Selects®

Serve with a spinach salad with Mandarin oranges and reduced-fat sweet and sour dressing and 1 toasted breadstick spread with 1 teaspoon light margarine.

Nutritional Information: 338 calories; 9g fat (22.5% calories from fat); 15g protein; 53g carbohydrate; 5g dietary fiber; 40mg cholesterol; 846mg sodium.

DAY 5

Breakfast

1 small (2 oz.) fat-free bran muffin
1 tsp. reduced-calorie margarine
1 tsp. peach jam

1/2 medium banana
1 cup plain nonfat yogurt

Nutritional Information: 382 calories; 9g fat (20.9% calories from fat); 18g protein; 59g carbohydrate; 3g dietary fiber; 26mg cholesterol; 485mg sodium.

Lunch

Skinless Roast Chicken Breast

2 oz. boneless, skinless roasted
   chicken breast
2/3 cup wide noodles

1 cup steamed broccoli (cooked with
   1 tsp. light margarine)

Serve with *Spinach Salad* and $3/4$ cup plain nonfat yogurt mixed with $1/2$ cup canned peach slices (no sugar added). Serves 1.

Spinach Salad

2 cups spinach leaves, torn	1 tbsp. imitation bacon bits
$1/2$ cup mushrooms, sliced	1 tbsp. fresh lemon juice
$1/2$ cup red onion	

Nutritional Information: 459 calories; 7g fat (13.9% calories from fat); 36g protein; 66g carbohydrate; 9g dietary fiber; 79mg cholesterol; 409mg sodium.

....

Dinner

Cajun Spiced Tilapia

3 tbsp. Tony Cachere Original Creole Seasoning®	$1^1/4$ lbs. (4 fillets) tilapia nonstick cooking spray

Spice tilapia liberally with Creole Seasoning. Heat skillet to medium-high heat and spray with nonstick cooking spray. Add spiced tilapia fillets and grill for 4 minutes on each side. Serve with 2 cups spring lettuce mixed with light Ranch dressing, 1 cup mashed potatoes and 1 dinner roll. Serves 4.

Nutritional Information: 375 calories; 8g fat (18.7% calories from fat); 33g protein; 43g carbohydrate; 6g dietary fiber; 66mg cholesterol; 725mg sodium.

DAY 6

....

Breakfast

$1^1/2$ cups puffed-wheat cereal	1 cup nonfat milk
1 large tangerine	

Nutritional Information: 225 calories; 1g fat (3.6% calories from fat); 12g protein; 45g carbohydrate; 5g dietary fiber; 4mg cholesterol; 129mg sodium.

....

Lunch

Grilled Ham, Muenster and Spinach Sandwiches

8 oz. thinly sliced lower-sodium deli ham	4 (1-oz.) slices reduced-sodium Muenster cheese

8 ($^3/_4$-oz.) slices crusty Chicago-style Italian bread (about $^1/_2$ inch thick), toasted
2 cups fresh baby spinach

1 tbsp. chowchow or sweet pickle relish
nonstick cooking spray

Layer each of 4 bread slices with 2 ounces ham, 1 slice Muenster cheese, $^1/_2$ cup baby spinach, 1 tablespoon chowchow and 1 bread slice. Heat a large nonstick skillet over medium-high heat. Coat sandwiches with cooking spray and add to pan. Cook 2 minutes on each side or until browned and cheese melts. Cut sandwiches in half, if desired. Serve immediately. Serves 4. (Note: Chowchow is a spicy sweet relish made from cucumbers, onions, peppers and other vegetables. Sweet pickle relish may be substituted if chowchow is not available in your area.)

Nutritional Information: 315 calories; 11g fat (33% calories from fat); 20.8g protein; 32.4g carbohydrate; 1.7g dietary fiber; 53mg cholesterol; 821mg sodium.

....

Dinner

Penne with Sage and Mushrooms

1 whole garlic head
2 tbsp. plus 1 tsp. olive oil
$2^1/_2$ cups boiling water, divided
$^1/_2$ oz. dried wild mushroom blend (about $^3/_4$ cup)
8 oz. uncooked whole-grain penne pasta
$^1/_4$ cup fresh sage leaves

$2^1/_2$ cups sliced mushrooms (about 6 oz.)
$^1/_2$ tsp. salt
$^1/_2$ tsp. freshly ground black pepper
1 cup fat-free, less-sodium chicken broth
2 oz. fresh Parmesan cheese, divided

Preheat oven to 400° F. Cut top off garlic head. Place in a small baking dish and drizzle with 1 teaspoon oil. Cover dish with foil and bake at 400° F for 45 minutes. Remove dish from oven. Add $^1/_2$ cup boiling water to dish then cover and let stand 30 minutes. Separate cloves and squeeze to extract garlic pulp into water. Discard skins. Mash garlic pulp mixture with a fork and set aside. Combine remaining 2 cups boiling water and dried mushrooms in a bowl. Cover and let stand 30 minutes. Rinse mushrooms, drain well and roughly chop. Set aside. Cook pasta according to package directions, omitting salt and fat. Heat remaining 2 tablespoons of oil in a large nonstick skillet over medium-high heat. Add sage to pan and sauté 1 minute or until crisp and browned. Remove from pan using a slotted spoon and set aside. Add mushrooms, salt and pepper to pan; sauté 4 minutes. Add garlic mixture, chopped mushrooms and broth to pan. Cook 5 minutes or until liquid is reduced by about half. Grate $1^1/_2$ ounces cheese. Stir pasta and grated cheese into pan. Cover and let stand 5 minutes. Thinly shave remaining $^1/_2$ ounce of cheese. Top each serving evenly with cheese shavings and sage leaves. Serves 4.

Nutritional Information: 350 calories; 13g fat (34% calories from fat); 14.6g protein; 51.1g carbohydrate; 7.8g dietary fiber; 9mg cholesterol; 550mg sodium.

DAY 7

Breakfast

1 cup Wheat Chex®   1 cup nonfat milk
1 banana, sliced

Nutritional Information: 363 calories; 2g fat (5% calories from fat); 14g protein; 77g carbohydrate; 7g dietary fiber; 4mg cholesterol; 436mg sodium.

Lunch

Honey-Gingered Carrot Soup & Smoked Turkey Sandwich

3 cups fat-free, less-sodium chicken   1 tbsp. minced peeled fresh ginger
   broth   1 tsp. grated orange rind
2 (10-oz.) pkg. frozen sliced honey- $^1/_4$ tsp. black pepper
   glazed carrots (such as Green   plain fat-free yogurt (optional)
   Giant), thawed   thyme sprigs (optional)
$^1/_2$ cup frozen chopped onion

Combine chicken broth, carrots, onion, ginger, orange rind and pepper in a large saucepan and bring to a boil. Reduce heat and simmer 2 minutes or until carrots are tender. Place half of soup mixture in a blender or food processor. Remove center piece of blender lid (to allow steam to escape); secure blender lid on blender. Place a clean towel over opening in blender lid (to avoid splatters). Blend 30 seconds or until smooth. Pour pureed mixture into a large bowl. Repeat procedure with remaining soup mixture. Ladle soup into bowls and garnish with yogurt and thyme sprigs, if desired. Serves 4.

Smoked Turkey Sandwich

2 slices whole-wheat bread
2 oz. sliced smoked turkey
1 tbsp. light mayonnaise

2 slices tomato
1 romaine lettuce leaf

Assemble and enjoy with *Honey-Gingered Carrot Soup*.

Nutritional Information: 394 calories; 9g fat (25% calories from fat); 19.7g protein; 53.7g carbohydrate; 7.8g dietary fiber; 31mg cholesterol; 1,211mg sodium.

Dinner

Butternut Squash Pizzas

1 cup thinly sliced onion
$1/2$ butternut squash, seeded and
thinly sliced
1 tsp. chopped fresh rosemary
salt and pepper to taste

1 tbsp. olive oil, divided
1 pkg. refrigerated pizza crust
1 tbsp. cornmeal
2 tbsp. grated Parmesan cheese

Preheat oven to 400° F. Place sliced onion and squash in a roasting pan. Sprinkle with rosemary, salt, pepper and 1 tablespoon of the olive oil; toss to coat. Bake in the preheated oven for 20 minutes, or until onions are lightly browned and squash is tender; set aside. Increase oven temperature to 450° F. On a floured surface, roll each ball of dough into an 8-inch round. Place the rounds on a baking sheet sprinkled with cornmeal (you may need 2 baking sheets depending on their size). Distribute squash mixture over the two rounds and continue baking for 10 minutes, checking occasionally, or until the crust is firm. Sprinkle with cheese and the remaining tablespoon olive oil. Cut into quarters, and serve.

Nutritional Information: 342 calories; 7g fat (17.6% calories from fat); 10g protein; 63g carbohydrate; 4g dietary fiber; 2mg cholesterol; 528mg sodium.

Second Week Grocery List

Produce
- [ ] apples
- [ ] avocados
- [ ] bananas
- [ ] berries
- [ ] blueberries
- [ ] carrots
- [ ] celery
- [ ] cherry tomatoes
- [ ] cilantro
- [ ] cucumbers
- [ ] garlic
- [ ] ginger
- [ ] green beans
- [ ] green onions
- [ ] honeydew melon
- [ ] jalapeño pepper
- [ ] lemons
- [ ] mixed veggies
- [ ] olives
- [ ] onions
- [ ] parsley
- [ ] potatoes
- [ ] red onion
- [ ] red peppers
- [ ] romaine lettuce
- [ ] spring mix
- [ ] strawberries
- [ ] tomatoes

Baking Products
- [ ] balsamic vinegar
- [ ] chili powder
- [ ] cinnamon
- [ ] cloves

- [ ] cumin
- [ ] Dijon mustard
- [ ] dried basil, whole
- [ ] dried oregano, whole
- [ ] dried red pepper, ground
- [ ] garlic powder
- [ ] ground pepper
- [ ] honey
- [ ] honey mustard
- [ ] ketchup
- [ ] kosher salt
- [ ] lime juice
- [ ] nonstick cooking spray
- [ ] nutmeg, ground
- [ ] olive oil
- [ ] paprika
- [ ] pepper, freshly ground black
- [ ] pesto
- [ ] Ranch salad dressing, light
- [ ] rosemary
- [ ] salad dressing, light
- [ ] salt
- [ ] soy sauce, reduced-sodium
- [ ] syrup, low-sugar
- [ ] Worcestershire sauce

Breads and Cereals
- [ ] baked tortilla chips
- [ ] bread, sourdough light
- [ ] bread, whole-wheat
- [ ] cornbread
- [ ] cornflakes
- [ ] corn tortillas
- [ ] dinner rolls, whole-wheat
- [ ] English muffins, whole-wheat

- ❑ farfalle (bow-tie pasta)
- ❑ French bread
- ❑ hoagie rolls
- ❑ manicotti
- ❑ pasta
- ❑ pretzel twists

Canned Foods
- ❑ beans chili (1 can)
- ❑ beef broth
- ❑ black beans (1 can)
- ❑ chipotle chili, canned in abodo sauce
- ❑ corn, no-salt-added whole-kernel (1 can)
- ❑ Mandarin oranges (1 can)
- ❑ minestrone soups, condensed (3 cans)
- ❑ refried beans, organic
- ❑ tomato paste (2 cans)
- ❑ tomatoes, stewed (1 can)
- ❑ tomatoes with green chiles (1 can)

Dairy Products
- ❑ Asiago cheese
- ❑ Cool Whip Lite®
- ❑ cottage cheese, lowfat

- ❑ eggs
- ❑ margarine, light
- ❑ milk, lowfat
- ❑ milk, nonfat
- ❑ Monterey Jack cheese
- ❑ Parmesan cheese
- ❑ sour cream, light
- ❑ Swiss cheese
- ❑ Yoplait Light Orange Crème® yogurt

Frozen Foods
- ❑ Lean Cuisine Casual Eating® frozen meal
- ❑ pancakes, lowfat
- ❑ spinach

Meat and Poultry
- ❑ chicken breasts, roasted skinless, boneless
- ❑ crab meat
- ❑ $1^1/_2$ lbs. ground beef, lean
- ❑ deli ham, reduced-fat
- ❑ deli roast beef
- ❑ 16 oz. lamb chops, lean
- ❑ (4) 4-oz. pork chops, boneless, center-cut loin
- ❑ trout, clean and boned

Second Week Meals and Recipes

DAY 1

Breakfast

2 frozen lowfat pancakes, heated
1 tbsp. low-sugar syrup
1 tsp. light margarine

2-inch wedge honeydew melon
1 cup nonfat milk

Nutritional Information: 375 calories; 5g fat (11.5% calories from fat); 13g protein; 71g carbohydrate; 2g dietary fiber; 11mg cholesterol; 556mg sodium.

Lunch

Lean Cuisine Casual Eating®
    frozen meal
2 cups tossed spring mix salad

1 cup berries with 2 tbsp. Cool
    Whip Lite®

Nutritional Information: 333 calories; 8g fat (19.7% calories from fat); 15g protein; 56g carbohydrate; 10g dietary fiber; 40mg cholesterol; 635mg sodium.

Dinner

Pasta with Sauce

$^2/_3$ cup light prepared pesto
(1) 8-oz. pkg. fresh pasta (9 oz.)
1 tbsp. olive oil
3 cloves garlic, minced

2 cups roasted red pepper
$^1/_2$ cup olives, pitted and halved
salt and pepper, to taste

Place the pesto in a large bowl. Cook the pasta according to package directions. While the pasta is cooking, heat the oil in a large skillet over medium-high heat. Add the garlic and cook, stirring until soft, about 30 seconds. Add the peppers and olives and cook, stirring until hot, about 3 minutes. Season with salt and pepper. Drain the cooked pasta, reserving $^1/_3$ cup of the water. Whisk the pasta water into the pesto. Add the pasta to the pesto and toss to combine. Add the peppers and olives and combine. Serve with 2 cups mixed greens, with diced tomato and cucumber and light dressing. Serves 4.

Nutritional Information: 260 calories; 7g fat (23.2% calories from fat); 9g protein; 43g carbohydrate; 7g dietary fiber; 41mg cholesterol; 168mg sodium.

DAY 2

....

Breakfast

Egg and Cheese Breakfast Tacos with Homemade Salsa

1 cup chopped tomato
$^1/_4$ cup chopped red onion
2 tbsp. chopped fresh cilantro
1 tsp. minced jalapeño pepper
$^1/_4$ tsp. kosher salt
4 tsp. fresh lime juice, divided
1 tsp. minced garlic, divided
1 cup organic refried beans
$^1/_4$ tsp. ground cumin

1 tbsp. 1-percent lowfat milk
6 large eggs, lightly beaten
$^1/_4$ cup chopped green onions
8 (6-inch) corn tortillas
$^1/_2$ cup (2 oz.) shredded Monterey
  Jack cheese with jalapeño peppers
8 tsp. reduced-fat sour cream
nonstick cooking spray

Combine the first 5 ingredients in a small bowl. Stir in 2 teaspoons lime juice and $^1/_2$ teaspoon garlic. Combine beans, remaining 2 teaspoons lime juice, remaining $^1/_2$ teaspoon garlic and cumin in another bowl. Combine milk and eggs in a medium bowl and stir with a whisk. Heat a large nonstick skillet over medium-high heat. Coat pan with cooking spray. Add green onions to pan and sauté 1 minute, stirring frequently. Stir in egg mixture. Cook 3 minutes or until soft-scrambled, stirring constantly. Remove from heat. Warm tortillas according to package directions. Spread 1 tablespoon bean mixture on each tortilla. Spoon about 2 tablespoons egg mixture down center of each tortilla. Top each serving with 1 tablespoon tomato mixture, 1 tablespoon cheese and 1 teaspoon sour cream. Serve with 1 cup of fresh mango. Serves 4.

Nutritional Information: 441 calories; 13.3g fat (26% calories from fat); 20g protein; 62g carbohydrate; 10.5g dietary fiber; 289mg cholesterol; 407mg sodium.

....

Lunch

French-style Grilled Ham and Cheese

4 ($1^1/_2$-oz.) slices French bread
4 tsp. honey mustard
6 oz. reduced-fat deli ham, thin sliced
$^1/_2$ cup nonfat milk

4 (1-ounce) slices reduced-fat
  Swiss cheese
3 large egg whites
nonstick cooking spray

Cut a slit in each bread slice to form a pocket. Spread 1 teaspoon honey mustard into each bread pocket. Divide ham and cheese evenly among bread pockets. Combine milk and egg whites in a shallow bowl, stirring with a whisk. Dip sandwiches, 1 at a time, in milk mixture, turning to coat. Heat a large nonstick skillet coated with cooking spray over medium-high heat. Add 2 sandwiches; cook 3 minutes on each side or until golden brown. Repeat procedure with remaining sandwiches. Serve with 1 cup berries with 2 tablespoons Cool Whip Lite® and 1 ounce pretzel twists. Serves 4.

Nutritional Information: 461 calories; 10.8g fat (22% calories from fat); 22.3g protein; 62g carbohydrate; 5.38g dietary fiber; 40mg cholesterol; 1,082mg sodium.

Dinner

Chili Soup

$1^1/_2$ pounds lean ground beef
3 cans minestrone soup, condensed (10-$^3/_4$ oz.)
1 can tomatoes, stewed ($14^1/_2$-oz.) diced

1 medium onion, chopped
1 can tomatoes with green chilies (10 oz.) diced
1 can beans ($15^1/_2$-oz.) chili
4 cups water

Brown together ground beef and chopped onion. Drain thoroughly. Add remaining ingredients and mix together. Simmer for 10 minutes. Serve with 2 cups spring mix salad with light Ranch dressing and one 2-inch cube of cornbread. Serves 12.

Nutritional Information: 438 calories; 18g fat (36.9% calories from fat); 21g protein; 48g carbohydrate; 5g dietary fiber; 69mg cholesterol; 1,018mg sodium.

DAY 3

Breakfast

1 small (2 oz.) whole-wheat English muffin, split and toasted
1 tsp. light margarine

1 cup sliced strawberries
$^1/_2$ cup nonfat milk

Nutritional Information: 224 calories; 4g fat (14.7% calories from fat); 10g protein; 41g carbohydrate; 7g dietary fiber; 2mg cholesterol; 472mg sodium.

Lunch

Chick-fil-A Chargrilled Chicken Sandwich®

fruit cup

Nutritional Information: 340 calories; 3.5g fat (14.7% calories from fat); 28g protein; 50g carbohydrate; 5g dietary fiber; 65mg cholesterol; 940mg sodium.

Dinner

Honey and Spice-glazed Pork Chops

$^1/_4$ cup honey
2 tbsp. Dijon mustard
$^1/_2$ tsp. ground ginger
$^1/_4$ tsp. ground cinnamon
$^1/_8$ tsp. ground cloves

4 (4-oz.) boneless center-cut loin
  pork chops (about $^1/_2$ inch thick)
$^1/_2$ tsp. salt
$^1/_4$ tsp. freshly ground black pepper
nonstick cooking spray

Combine first 5 ingredients in a bowl. Heat a large nonstick skillet coated with cooking spray over medium-high heat. Sprinkle pork with salt and pepper and cook 2 minutes on each side or until browned. Reduce heat to medium-low and add honey mixture. Cook 10 minutes or until done, turning pork once. Serve with $^1/_2$ cup mashed potatoes and 1 cup steamed green beans. Serves 4.

Nutritional Information: 438 calories; 14.1g fat (29% calories from fat); 38g protein; 40.7g carbohydrate; 6.3g dietary fiber; 94mg cholesterol; 869mg sodium.

DAY 4

Breakfast

$^1/_2$ cup cornflakes cereal
2 slices whole-wheat bread, toasted
1 tsp. light margarine

$^1/_2$ medium banana, sliced
1 cup nonfat milk

Nutritional Information: 345 calories; 5g fat (12.5% calories from fat); 15g protein; 64g carbohydrate; 6g dietary fiber; 4mg cholesterol; 617mg sodium.

Lunch

Spicy Bistro Steak Subs

1 tbsp. stick margarine
2 garlic cloves, minced
1 lb. thinly sliced lean deli roast beef
2 tbsp. ketchup
4 tsp. Worcestershire sauce
$^1/_2$ tsp. dried basil

$^1/_2$ tsp. dried oregano
$^1/_4$ tsp. ground red pepper
$1^1/_2$ cups beef broth
6 ($2^1/_2$-oz.) hoagie rolls with sesame
  seeds, cut in half lengthwise
carrot curls and olives (optional)

Melt margarine in a large nonstick skillet over medium-high heat. Add minced garlic, and sauté 2 minutes. Add roast beef and the next 6 ingredients (roast beef through broth) and bring to a boil. Reduce heat and simmer

2 minutes, stirring frequently. Drain roast beef in a colander over a bowl, reserving sauce. Divide roast beef evenly among roll bottoms, and top with roll tops. Serve sandwiches with reserved sauce. Garnish sandwiches with carrot curls and olives, if desired. Serve with 1 apple. Serves 6.

Nutritional Information: 426 calories; 10.6g fat (4.9% calories from fat); 21.4g protein; 61.6g carbohydrate; 5.6g dietary fiber; 2mg cholesterol; 938 sodium.

....

Dinner

Spinach Manicotti

10 manicotti	$1/_4$ tsp. pepper
2 cans tomato paste (6 oz.)	2 pkg. frozen chopped spinach (10 oz.)
3 cups water	1 ctn. cottage cheese, lowfat (16 oz.)
$1/_2$ onion, finely chopped	$1/_3$ cup Parmesan cheese, grated
2 cloves garlic, crushed	$1/_4$ tsp. ground nutmeg
$1/_2$ tsp. dried whole basil	pepper (to taste)
$1/_2$ tsp. dried whole oregano	1 tsp. fresh parsley, chopped
$1/_4$ tsp. salt	nonstick cooking spray

Cook manicotti shells according to package directions, omitting salt; drain and set aside. Combine next 8 ingredients and cover and cook sauce over low heat for 1 hour. Cook spinach according to package directions, omitting salt. Drain and place on paper towel and squeeze until barely moist. Combine spinach, cottage cheese, Parmesan cheese and nutmeg. Stuff manicotti shells with spinach mixture and arrange in a 13" x 9" x 2" baking dish coated with nonstick cooking spray. Pour tomato sauce over manicotti. Bake at 350° F for 45 minutes. Garnish with parsley. Serve with 2-inch French bread slice and 2 cups tossed salad with 2 tablespoons light Ranch dressing. Serves 5.

Nutritional Information: 516 calories; 6g fat (9.8% calories from fat); 33g protein; 87g carbohydrate; 13g dietary fiber; 8mg cholesterol; 1,538mg sodium.

DAY 5

....

Breakfast

2 slices light sourdough bread	$3/_4$ cup blueberries
1 tsp. light margarine	1 cup nonfat milk

Nutritional Information: 300 calories; 4g fat (12.4% calories from fat); 13g protein; 53g carbohydrate; 4g dietary fiber; 4mg cholesterol; 483mg sodium.

Lunch

McDonald's Premium Southwest Salad with Grilled Chicken®

¹/₂ packet of Balsamic Vinaigrette
1 apple

Nutritional Information: 401 calories; 8g fat (25% calories from fat); 30g protein; 51g carbohydrate; 10g dietary fiber; 70mg cholesterol; 960mg sodium.

Dinner

Savory Lamb Chops

2 tbsp. Dijon mustard
2 tbsp. fresh rosemary or 2 tsp. dried rosemary, crushed

2 tsp. honey
¹/₂ tsp. coarsely ground pepper
16 oz. lamb chop, lean (4-oz.)

Preheat grill to medium-high heat. Combine first 4 ingredients in a small bowl and stir well. Trim fat from lamb and place chops on the grill. Grill 5 minutes on each side. Brush mustard mixture over chops. Broil chops 2 minutes on each side or until desired degree of doneness, basting occasionally with mustard mixture. Serve with 1 cup steamed mixed vegetables and 1 whole-wheat dinner roll. Serves 4.

Nutritional Information: 484 calories; 13g fat (23.9% calories from fat); 30g protein; 64g carbohydrate; 11g dietary fiber; 63mg cholesterol; 937mg sodium.

DAY 6

Breakfast

Carole's Breakfast Surprise

(1) 6-oz. carton Yoplait Light Orange Crème® yogurt
¹/₄ cup cottage cheese

4-oz. can Mandarin oranges (drained)
1 tbsp. Cool Whip Lite®

Mix all ingredients and enjoy.

Nutritional Information: 185 calories; 1g fat (6.6% calories from fat); 16g protein; 27g carbohydrate; 2g dietary fiber; 7mg cholesterol; 337mg sodium.

Lunch

Chipotle Chicken Taco Salad

2 cups chopped roasted skinless, boneless chicken breasts

1 cup cherry tomatoes, halved
4 cups shredded romaine lettuce

$^1/_3$ cup thinly vertically sliced red
  onion
(1) 15-oz. can black beans, rinsed and
  drained

$^1/_2$ cup diced peeled avocado
(1) 8$^3/_4$-oz. can no-salt-added
  whole-kernel corn, rinsed
  and drained

Dressing

$^1/_3$ cup chopped fresh cilantro
$^2/_3$ cup light sour cream
1 tbsp. minced chipotle chile, canned
  in adobo sauce

1 tsp. ground cumin
1 tsp. chili powder
4 tsp. fresh lime juice
$^1/_4$ tsp. salt

To prepare dressing, combine first 7 ingredients, stirring well. To prepare salad, combine lettuce and remaining ingredients in a large bowl. Drizzle dressing over salad and toss gently to coat. Serve immediately. Serve with 1 ounce of baked tortilla chips. Serves 4. (Tip: Add a spoonful of adobo sauce for a spicier salad. Kidney or pinto beans also taste great in this dish.)

Nutritional Information: 360 calories; 9.2g fat (14.2% calories from fat); 26.3g protein; 47.1g carbohydrate; 9g dietary fiber; 50mg cholesterol; 862mg sodium.

Dinner

Crab-stuffed Trout

2 whole trout (6 oz.) cleaned and
  boned
3 tsp. reduced-sodium soy sauce,
  divided
3 oz. crab meat, shredded
2 slices bread
$^1/_2$ cup carrots, shredded

$^1/_4$ cup celery, thinly sliced
$^1/_4$ cup green onion, thinly sliced
1 egg white, slightly beaten
1 tbsp. lemon peel, grated
1 tsp. garlic powder
$^1/_2$ tsp. ground black pepper
lemon wedges

Preheat oven to 375° F. Wash trout and pat dry with paper towels. Place on foil-lined baking sheet. Brush inside cavities lightly with one-half the soy sauce. Combine remaining soy sauce, crab meat, bread crumbs, carrots, celery, onion, egg white, lemon peel, garlic powder and pepper in a small bowl. Place one-half the stuffing inside each trout. Bake 30 minutes. Serve with lemon wedges. Serve with *Baked Fries* recipe below and 1 slice French bread. Serves 4.

Nutritional Information: 563 calories; 9g fat (14.2% calories from fat); 35g protein; 85g carbohydrate; 7g dietary fiber; 68mg cholesterol; 828mg sodium.

Baked Fries

(1) 3-oz. baking potato, cut thin $^1/_4$ tsp. paprika
$^1/_4$ tsp. salt   nonstick cooking spray

Preheat oven to 450° F. Place potato sticks onto a nonstick baking sheet and spray sticks lightly with nonstick cooking spray. Sprinkle sticks with salt and paprika and bake for 10-12 minutes or until crispy outside and tender inside.

Nutritional Information: 69 calories; trace fat (2% calories from fat); 2g protein; 16g carbohydrate; 1g dietary fiber; 0mg cholesterol; 538mg sodium.

DAY 7

....

Breakfast

1 small (2 oz.) bagel $^3/_4$ cup artificially sweetened mixed-
1 tsp. strawberry all-fruit spread   berry nonfat yogurt
$^3/_4$ cup blackberries

Nutritional Information: 314 calories; 2g fat (4.5% calories from fat); 14g protein; 62g carbohydrate; 8g dietary fiber; 2mg cholesterol; 404mg sodium.

....

Lunch

Warm Bow-Tie Pasta Salad

8 oz. uncooked farfalle (bow-tie   3 tbsp. balsamic vinegar
  pasta)   1 tbsp. Dijon mustard
2 tbsp. olive oil, divided $^1/_4$ tsp. salt
1$^1/_3$ cups julienne-cut red bell pepper   6 cups gourmet salad greens
  (about 1 large pepper) $^1/_2$ cup (2 oz.) finely grated Asiago
1 cup sliced mushrooms (about 2   cheese
  ounces)   freshly ground black pepper
3 garlic cloves, minced   (optional)

Cook the pasta according to the package directions, omitting the salt and fat. While the pasta is cooking, heat 1 tablespoon oil in a large nonstick skillet over medium heat. Add bell pepper, mushrooms and garlic and sauté for 10 minutes. Combine 1 tablespoon oil, vinegar, mustard and salt in a large bowl. Drain pasta. Add pasta, salad greens and mushroom mixture to bowl and toss well. Serve with cheese and black pepper, if desired. Serves 4.

Nutritional Information: 360 calories; 12.1g fat (30% calories from fat); 14.1g protein; 48.6g carbohydrate; 3.6g dietary fiber; 15mg cholesterol; 441mg sodium.

Dinner

2 Taco Bell Chicken Soft Tacos Fresco Style®

2 cups mixed green salad served with 2 tbsp. light Ranch dressing

Nutritional Information: 471 calories; 20g fat (38.7% calories from fat); 25g protein; 48g carbohydrate; 10g dietary fiber; 50mg cholesterol; 1,197mg sodium.

DESSERT RECIPES

(**Note:** Add the ingredients for each of these items to the grocery lists.)

Spanish Style Peach Pie

(4) 6″ flour tortillas
(3) fresh peaches, halved, with pits removed
$1/4$ cup light margarine, melted
juice of 1 large lemon

$1/2$ cup brown sugar or calorie-free sweetener
1 tsp. almond extract

Heat oven to 350° F. Spray eight 6-oz. baking dishes with nonstick cooking spray. Fold each tortilla in half and arrange in one of the prepared baking dishes. Set aside. Spray vegetable grilling rack or basket with nonstick cooking spray. Arrange peaches cut side down on rack or basket. Grill for five minutes on each side. Slice peaches and combine with butter, $1/4$ cup brown sugar, lemon juice and almond extract in a saucepan and heat on medium low for five minutes. Fill each tortilla-lined baking dish with peach mixture and sprinkle with remaining brown sugar or sugar replacement. Place individual dishes on a baking sheet and bake for 15 minutes or until golden brown. Serves 4.

Nutritional Information: 192 calories; 5g fat (22.6% calories from fat); trace protein; 36g carbohydrate; 3g dietary fiber; 0mg cholesterol; 317mg sodium.

Banana Coconut Custard

3 eggs
3 bananas, cut in pieces
$1^1/2$ cups skim milk
1 cup coconut
$1/3$ cup flour, all-purpose

$1/2$ tsp. baking powder
$1/2$ tsp. nutmeg
$1/2$ tsp. vanilla extract
$1/4$ tsp. cinnamon

Blend eggs and bananas together in blender until smooth. Add remaining ingredients and blend. Pour into six 8-oz. custard cups. Preheat oven to 350° F. Place cups in a pan with one inch of water. Bake for 45 minutes or until custards are set. Refrigerate and serve. Serves 6.

Nutritional Information: 188 calories; 7g fat (34.7% calories from fat); 7g protein; 25g carbohydrate; 3g dietary fiber; 107mg cholesterol; 111mg sodium.

Easy Blueberry Tarts

2 tbsp. sugar
1 tsp. cornstarch
1/8 tsp. cayenne pepper
1/4 cup water
1 cup fresh blueberries
1 cup fresh raspberries

1 tbsp. sugar
1/4 tsp. ground cinnamon
4 sheets frozen phyllo dough
   (9" x 14" rectangles), thawed
nonstick cooking spray

Preheat oven to 375° F. Lightly coat four 4" x 2" x 1/2" rectangular tart pans that have removable bottoms with cooking spray and set aside. In a small saucepan, stir together 2 tablespoons sugar, the cornstarch and cayenne pepper. Stir in water and half of the blueberries. Cook and stir over medium heat until mixture is thickened and bubbly. Fold in remaining blueberries and the raspberries; set aside. In small bowl, stir together 1 tablespoon sugar and the cinnamon. Place one sheet of phyllo on cutting board. Lightly coat with cooking spray; sprinkle with about 1 teaspoon sugar mixture. Repeat layering with remaining phyllo and sugar mixture, ending with cooking spray. With a sharp knife, cut phyllo stack in half lengthwise and crosswise, forming four rectangles. Ease rectangles into prepared tart pans. Bake for 8 minutes or until phyllo is golden brown. Cool slightly and remove shells from pans. Spoon filling into shells just before serving. Serve warm or cool. Serves 4.

Nutritional Information: 131 calories; 1g fat; 2g protein; 29g carbohydrate, 3g dietary fiber; 93mg sodium.

SNACK RECIPES

(**Note:** Add the ingredients for each of these items to the grocery lists.)

Apple Raisin Crunch

4 red delicious apples
1/4 cup raisins
I Can't Believe It's Not Butter® spray
1/2 cup Splenda®

1 tbsp. cinnamon
1/4 cup Cheerios®
nonstick cooking spray

Spray a 13" x 9" pan with cooking spray. Lay cored, sliced apples in bottom of pan and spread raisins on top of apples. Spray apples and raisins with Butter Spray. Sprinkle with Splenda® and ground cinnamon. Sprinkle Cheerios® cereal over all and bake 30 minutes in the oven at 350° F. Serves 4.

Nutritional Information: 168 calories; 1g fat (3.5% calories from fat); 1g protein; 42g carbohydrate; 5g dietary fiber; 0mg cholesterol; 67mg sodium.

Banana Cream Pie Smoothie

1 cup sliced ripe banana
(about 1 large)
1 cup vanilla lowfat yogurt
$^1/_2$ cup 1-percent lowfat milk
1 tbsp. nonfat dry milk

2 tbsp. whole-wheat graham cracker
crumbs
$^1/_2$ tsp. vanilla extract
3 ice cubes (about $^1/_4$ cup)

Arrange banana slices in a single layer on a baking sheet and freeze until firm (about 1 hour). Place frozen banana and remaining ingredients in a blender. Process until smooth. Sprinkle with graham cracker crumbs. Serve immediately. Serves 2.

Nutritional Information: 216 calories; 2.8g fat (12% calories from fat); 9.8g protein; 39.3g carbohydrate; 1.9g dietary fiber; 9mg cholesterol; 145mg sodium.

Veggie Piglets in Blankets with Dipping Sauce

1 (8-oz.) package reduced-fat crescent
roll dough
16 meatless breakfast links

$^3/_4$ cup honey
$^1/_4$ cup Dijon mustard

Preheat oven to 375° F. Unroll dough and divide along perforations into triangles. Cut each dough triangle in half to form 2 triangles. Wrap one dough triangle around center of each breakfast link, starting at wide end of triangle. Arrange wrapped breakfast links on a baking sheet. Bake at 375° F for 15 minutes or until browned. Combine honey and mustard and serve with piglets. Serves 8. (Tip: Great for parties and a kid favorite.)

Nutritional Information: 227 calories; 8.2g fat (30.6% calories from fat); trace protein; 44.2g carbohydrate; 2.2g dietary fiber; 0mg cholesterol; 754mg sodium.

HEALTHY SNACK OPTIONS
(**Note:** Add the ingredients for each of these items to the grocery lists.)

- 4 cups light butter popcorn
- Fruit and fruit smoothies (combine $^1/_2$ cup lowfat yogurt, 1 cup berries, handful of ice and $^1/_4$ cup orange juice)
- Nonfat yogurt with fresh fruit and $^1/_4$ cup low-fat granola
- 100-percent frozen fruit bar
- 1 cup of your favorite low-sugar cereal
- 30 small pretzel sticks
- 1 banana-chocolate whip (combine 1 cup fat-free milk, 1 small banana, a squeeze of chocolate syrup and a handful of ice cubes in a blender)
- snack plate (25 red grapes, 3 tablespoons feta cheese and 6 crackers)

Member Survey

Please answer the following questions to help your leader plan your First Place 4 Health meetings so that your needs might be met in this session. Give this form to your leader at the first group meeting.

Name _____ Birth date _____

Please list those who live in your household.

Name	Relationship	Age

What church do you attend? _____

Are you interested in receiving more information about our church?

      Yes   No

Occupation _____

What talent or area of expertise would you be willing to share with our class?

_____

Why did you join First Place 4 Health?

_____

With notice, would you be willing to lead a Bible study discussion one week?

      Yes   No

Are you comfortable praying out loud? _____

If the assistant leader were absent, would you be willing to assist in weighing in members and possibly evaluating the Live It Trackers?

      Yes   No

Any other comments:

_____

_____

Personal Weight and Measurement Record

Week	Weight	+ or -	Goal this Session	Pounds to goal
1				
2				
3				
4				
5				
6				
7				
8				
9				
10				
11				
12				

Beginning Measurements

Waist _____ Hips _____ Thighs _____ Chest _____

Ending Measurements

Waist _____ Hips _____ Thighs _____ Chest _____

First Place 4 Health
Prayer Partner

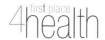

GOD'S PURPOSE
FOR YOU
Week
5

SCRIPTURE VERSE TO MEMORIZE FOR WEEK SIX:

*His divine power has given us everything we need for life and godliness
through our knowledge of him who called us by his own glory and goodness.*

2 PETER 1:3

Date: _____

Name: _____

Home Phone: (_____) _____

Work Phone: (_____) _____

Email: _____

Personal Prayer Concerns:

_____

_____

_____

_____

_____

_____

_____

This form is for prayer requests that are personal to you and your journey in First Place 4 Health. Please complete this form and have it ready to turn in when you arrive at your group meeting.

First Place 4 Health
Prayer Partner

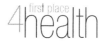

GOD'S PURPOSE
FOR YOU
Week
8

SCRIPTURE VERSE TO MEMORIZE FOR WEEK NINE:

Whether you turn to the right or to the left, your ears will hear a voice behind you, saying, "This is the way; walk in it."

ISAIAH 30:21

Date: _____

Name: _____

Home Phone: ( ) _____

Work Phone: ( ) _____

Email: _____

Personal Prayer Concerns:

_____

_____

_____

_____

_____

_____

_____

This form is for prayer requests that are personal to you and your journey in First Place 4 Health. Please complete this form and have it ready to turn in when you arrive at your group meeting.

First Place 4 Health
Prayer Partner

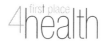

GOD'S PURPOSE
FOR YOU
Week
10

SCRIPTURE VERSE TO MEMORIZE FOR WEEK ELEVEN:

But you are a chosen people, a royal priesthood, a holy nation,
a people belonging to God, that you may declare the praises
of him who called you out of darkness into his wonderful light.

1 PETER 2:9

Date: _____

Name: _____

Home Phone: ( ) _____

Work Phone: ( ) _____

Email: _____

Personal Prayer Concerns:

_____

_____

_____

_____

_____

_____

_____

This form is for prayer requests that are personal to you and your journey in First Place 4 Health. Please complete this form and have it ready to turn in when you arrive at your group meeting.

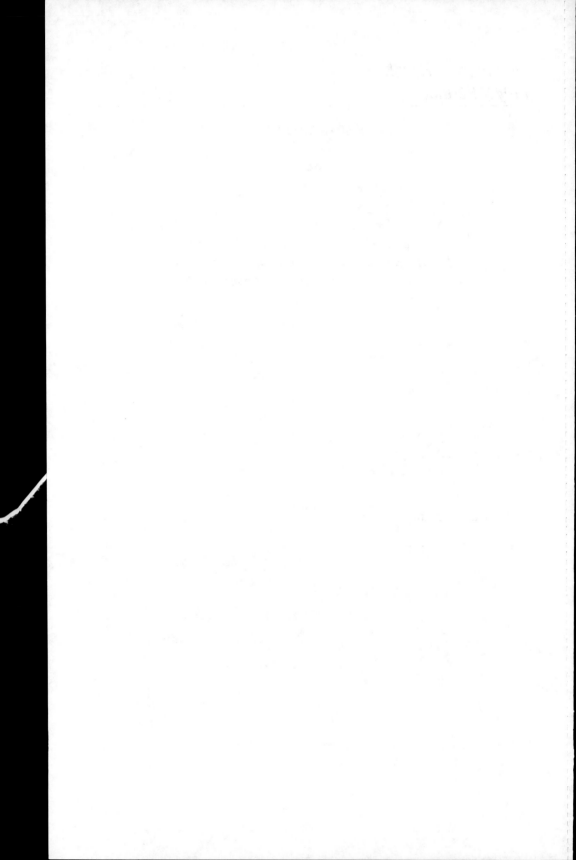

Live It Tracker

Name: _____ Loss/gain: _____ lbs.

Date: _____ Week #: _____ Calorie Range: _____ My food goal for next week: _____

Activity Level: None, < 30 min/day, 30-60 min/day, 60+ min/day My activity goal for next week: _____

Group	Daily Calories							
	1300-1400	1500-1600	1700-1800	1900-2000	2100-2200	2300-2400	2500-2600	2700-2800
Fruits	1.5-2 c.	1.5-2 c.	1.5-2 c.	2-2.5 c.	2-2.5 c.	2.5-3.5 c.	3.5-4.5 c.	3.5-4.5 c.
Vegetables	1.5-2 c.	2-2.5 c.	2.5-3 c.	2.5-3 c.	3-3.5 c.	3.5-4.5 c.	4.5-5 c.	4.5-5 c.
Grains	5 oz-eq.	5-6 oz-eq.	6-7 oz-eq.	6-7 oz-eq.	7-8 oz-eq.	8-9 oz-eq.	9-10 oz-eq.	10-11 oz-eq.
Meat & Beans	4 oz-eq.	5 oz-eq.	5-5.5 oz-eq.	5.5-6.5 oz-eq.	6.5-7 oz-eq.	7-7.5 oz-eq.	7-7.5 oz-eq.	7.5-8 oz-eq.
Milk	2-3 c.	3 c.	3 c.	3 c.	3 c.	3 c.	3 c.	3 c.
Healthy Oils	4 tsp.	5 tsp.	5 tsp.	6 tsp.	6 tsp.	7 tsp.	8 tsp.	8 tsp.

Day/Date:

Breakfast: _____   Lunch: _____

Dinner: _____   Snack: _____

Group	Fruits	Vegetables	Grains	Meat & Beans	Milk	Oils
Goal Amount						
Estimate Your Total						
Increase ⇧ or Decrease? ⇩						

Physical Activity: _____   Spiritual Activity: _____

Steps/Miles/Minutes: _____

Day/Date:

Breakfast: _____   Lunch: _____

Dinner: _____   Snack: _____

Group	Fruits	Vegetables	Grains	Meat & Beans	Milk	Oils
Goal Amount						
Estimate Your Total						
Increase ⇧ or Decrease? ⇩						

Physical Activity: _____   Spiritual Activity: _____

Steps/Miles/Minutes: _____

Day/Date:

Breakfast: _____   Lunch: _____

Dinner: _____   Snack: _____

Group	Fruits	Vegetables	Grains	Meat & Beans	Milk	Oils
Goal Amount						
Estimate Your Total						
Increase ⇧ or Decrease? ⇩						

Physical Activity: _____   Spiritual Activity: _____

Steps/Miles/Minutes: _____

Day/Date:

Breakfast: _____ Lunch: _____

Dinner: _____ Snack: _____

Group	Fruits	Vegetables	Grains	Meat & Beans	Milk	Oils
Goal Amount						
Estimate Your Total						
Increase ⇧ or Decrease? ⇩						

Physical Activity: _____ Spiritual Activity: _____

Steps/Miles/Minutes: _____ _____

Day/Date:

Breakfast: _____ Lunch: _____

Dinner: _____ Snack: _____

Group	Fruits	Vegetables	Grains	Meat & Beans	Milk	Oils
Goal Amount						
Estimate Your Total						
Increase ⇧ or Decrease? ⇩						

Physical Activity: _____ Spiritual Activity: _____

Steps/Miles/Minutes: _____ _____

Day/Date:

Breakfast: _____ Lunch: _____

Dinner: _____ Snack: _____

Group	Fruits	Vegetables	Grains	Meat & Beans	Milk	Oils
Goal Amount						
Estimate Your Total						
Increase ⇧ or Decrease? ⇩						

Physical Activity: _____ Spiritual Activity: _____

Steps/Miles/Minutes: _____ _____

Day/Date:

Breakfast: _____ Lunch: _____

Dinner: _____ Snack: _____

Group	Fruits	Vegetables	Grains	Meat & Beans	Milk	Oils
Goal Amount						
Estimate Your Total						
Increase ⇧ or Decrease? ⇩						

Physical Activity: _____ Spiritual Activity: _____

Steps/Miles/Minutes: _____ _____

Live It Tracker

Name: _____ Loss/gain: _____ lbs.

Date: _____ Week #: _____ Calorie Range: _____ My food goal for next week: _____

Activity Level: None, < 30 min/day, 30-60 min/day, 60+ min/day My activity goal for next week: _____

Group	Daily Calories							
	1300-1400	1500-1600	1700-1800	1900-2000	2100-2200	2300-2400	2500-2600	2700-2800
Fruits	1.5-2 c.	1.5-2 c.	1.5-2 c.	2-2.5 c.	2-2.5 c.	2.5-3.5 c.	3.5-4.5 c.	3.5-4.5 c.
Vegetables	1.5-2 c.	2-2.5 c.	2.5-3 c.	2.5-3 c.	3-3.5 c.	3.5-4.5 c.	4.5-5 c.	4.5-5 c.
Grains	5 oz-eq.	5-6 oz-eq.	6-7 oz-eq.	6-7 oz-eq.	7-8 oz-eq.	8-9 oz-eq.	9-10 oz-eq.	10-11 oz-eq.
Meat & Beans	4 oz-eq.	5 oz-eq.	5-5.5 oz-eq.	5.5-6.5 oz-eq.	6.5-7 oz-eq.	7-7.5 oz-eq.	7-7.5 oz-eq.	7.5-8 oz-eq.
Milk	2-3 c.	3 c.	3 c.	3 c.	3 c.	3 c.	3 c.	3 c.
Healthy Oils	4 tsp.	5 tsp.	5 tsp.	6 tsp.	6 tsp.	7 tsp.	8 tsp.	8 tsp.

Day/Date:

Breakfast: _____ Lunch: _____

Dinner: _____ Snack: _____

Group	Fruits	Vegetables	Grains	Meat & Beans	Milk	Oils
Goal Amount						
Estimate Your Total						
Increase ⇧ or Decrease? ⇩						

Physical Activity: _____ Spiritual Activity: _____

Steps/Miles/Minutes: _____

Breakfast: _____ Lunch: _____

Dinner: _____ Snack: _____

Group	Fruits	Vegetables	Grains	Meat & Beans	Milk	Oils
Goal Amount						
Estimate Your Total						
Increase ⇧ or Decrease? ⇩						

Physical Activity: _____ Spiritual Activity: _____

Steps/Miles/Minutes: _____

Day/Date:

Breakfast: _____ Lunch: _____

Dinner: _____ Snack: _____

Group	Fruits	Vegetables	Grains	Meat & Beans	Milk	Oils
Goal Amount						
Estimate Your Total						
Increase ⇧ or Decrease? ⇩						

Physical Activity: _____ Spiritual Activity: _____

Steps/Miles/Minutes: _____

Day/Date:

Breakfast: _____ Lunch: _____

Dinner: _____ Snack: _____

Group	Fruits	Vegetables	Grains	Meat & Beans	Milk	Oils
Goal Amount						
Estimate Your Total						
Increase ⇧ or Decrease? ⇩						

Physical Activity: _____ Spiritual Activity: _____

Steps/Miles/Minutes: _____

Day/Date:

Breakfast: _____ Lunch: _____

Dinner: _____ Snack: _____

Group	Fruits	Vegetables	Grains	Meat & Beans	Milk	Oils
Goal Amount						
Estimate Your Total						
Increase ⇧ or Decrease? ⇩						

Physical Activity: _____ Spiritual Activity: _____

Steps/Miles/Minutes: _____

Day/Date:

Breakfast: _____ Lunch: _____

Dinner: _____ Snack: _____

Group	Fruits	Vegetables	Grains	Meat & Beans	Milk	Oils
Goal Amount						
Estimate Your Total						
Increase ⇧ or Decrease? ⇩						

Physical Activity: _____ Spiritual Activity: _____

Steps/Miles/Minutes: _____

Day/Date:

Breakfast: _____ Lunch: _____

Dinner: _____ Snack: _____

Group	Fruits	Vegetables	Grains	Meat & Beans	Milk	Oils
Goal Amount						
Estimate Your Total						
Increase ⇧ or Decrease? ⇩						

Physical Activity: _____ Spiritual Activity: _____

Steps/Miles/Minutes: _____

Live It Tracker

Name: _____ Loss/gain: _____ lbs.

Date: _____ Week #: ____ Calorie Range: _____ My food goal for next week: _____

Activity Level: None, < 30 min/day, 30-60 min/day, 60+ min/day My activity goal for next week: _____

Group	Daily Calories							
	1300-1400	1500-1600	1700-1800	1900-2000	2100-2200	2300-2400	2500-2600	2700-2800
Fruits	1.5-2 c.	1.5-2 c.	1.5-2 c.	2-2.5 c.	2-2.5 c.	2.5-3.5 c.	3.5-4.5 c.	3.5-4.5 c.
Vegetables	1.5-2 c.	2-2.5 c.	2.5-3 c.	2.5-3 c.	3-3.5 c.	3.5-4.5 c.	4.5-5 c.	4.5-5 c.
Grains	5 oz-eq.	5-6 oz-eq.	6-7 oz-eq.	6-7 oz-eq.	7-8 oz-eq.	8-9 oz-eq.	9-10 oz-eq.	10-11 oz-eq.
Meat & Beans	4 oz-eq.	5 oz-eq.	5-5.5 oz-eq.	5.5-6.5 oz-eq.	6.5-7 oz-eq.	7-7.5 oz-eq.	7-7.5 oz-eq.	7.5-8 oz-eq.
Milk	2-3 c.	3 c.	3 c.	3 c.	3 c.	3 c.	3 c.	3 c.
Healthy Oils	4 tsp.	5 tsp.	5 tsp.	6 tsp.	6 tsp.	7 tsp.	8 tsp.	8 tsp.

Day/Date:

Breakfast: _____ Lunch: _____

Dinner: _____ Snack: _____

Group	Fruits	Vegetables	Grains	Meat & Beans	Milk	Oils
Goal Amount						
Estimate Your Total						
Increase ⇧ or Decrease? ⇩						

Physical Activity: _____ Spiritual Activity: _____

Steps/Miles/Minutes: _____

Day/Date:

Breakfast: _____ Lunch: _____

Dinner: _____ Snack: _____

Group	Fruits	Vegetables	Grains	Meat & Beans	Milk	Oils
Goal Amount						
Estimate Your Total						
Increase ⇧ or Decrease? ⇩						

Physical Activity: _____ Spiritual Activity: _____

Steps/Miles/Minutes: _____

Day/Date:

Breakfast: _____ Lunch: _____

Dinner: _____ Snack: _____

Group	Fruits	Vegetables	Grains	Meat & Beans	Milk	Oils
Goal Amount						
Estimate Your Total						
Increase ⇧ or Decrease? ⇩						

Physical Activity: _____ Spiritual Activity: _____

Steps/Miles/Minutes: _____

Day/Date: ___

Breakfast: _____   Lunch: _____

Dinner: _____   Snack: _____
_____   _____

Group	Fruits	Vegetables	Grains	Meat & Beans	Milk	Oils
Goal Amount						
Estimate Your Total						
Increase ⇧ or Decrease? ⇩						

Physical Activity: _____   Spiritual Activity: _____

Steps/Miles/Minutes: _____   _____

Day/Date: ___

Breakfast: _____   Lunch: _____

Dinner: _____   Snack: _____
_____   _____

Group	Fruits	Vegetables	Grains	Meat & Beans	Milk	Oils
Goal Amount						
Estimate Your Total						
Increase ⇧ or Decrease? ⇩						

Physical Activity: _____   Spiritual Activity: _____

Steps/Miles/Minutes: _____   _____

Day/Date: ___

Breakfast: _____   Lunch: _____

Dinner: _____   Snack: _____
_____   _____

Group	Fruits	Vegetables	Grains	Meat & Beans	Milk	Oils
Goal Amount						
Estimate Your Total						
Increase ⇧ or Decrease? ⇩						

Physical Activity: _____   Spiritual Activity: _____

Steps/Miles/Minutes: _____   _____

Day/Date: ___

Breakfast: _____   Lunch: _____

Dinner: _____   Snack: _____
_____   _____

Group	Fruits	Vegetables	Grains	Meat & Beans	Milk	Oils
Goal Amount						
Estimate Your Total						
Increase ⇧ or Decrease? ⇩						

Physical Activity: _____   Spiritual Activity: _____

Steps/Miles/Minutes: _____   _____

Live It Tracker

Name: _____ Loss/gain: _____ lbs.

Date: _____ Week #: _____ Calorie Range: _____ My food goal for next week: _____

Activity Level: None, < 30 min/day, 30-60 min/day, 60+ min/day   My activity goal for next week: _____

Group	Daily Calories							
	1300-1400	1500-1600	1700-1800	1900-2000	2100-2200	2300-2400	2500-2600	2700-2800
Fruits	1.5-2 c.	1.5-2 c.	1.5-2 c.	2-2.5 c.	2-2.5 c.	2.5-3.5 c.	3.5-4.5 c.	3.5-4.5 c.
Vegetables	1.5-2 c.	2-2.5 c.	2.5-3 c.	2.5-3 c.	3-3.5 c.	3.5-4.5 c.	4.5-5 c.	4.5-5 c.
Grains	5 oz-eq.	5-6 oz-eq.	6-7 oz-eq.	6-7 oz-eq.	7-8 oz-eq.	8-9 oz-eq.	9-10 oz-eq.	10-11 oz-eq.
Meat & Beans	4 oz-eq.	5 oz-eq.	5-5.5 oz-eq.	5.5-6.5 oz-eq.	6.5-7 oz-eq.	7-7.5 oz-eq.	7-7.5 oz-eq.	7.5-8 oz-eq.
Milk	2-3 c.	3 c.	3 c.	3 c.	3 c.	3 c.	3 c.	3 c.
Healthy Oils	4 tsp.	5 tsp.	5 tsp.	6 tsp.	6 tsp.	7 tsp.	8 tsp.	8 tsp.

Day/Date: _____

Breakfast: _____   Lunch: _____

Dinner: _____   Snack: _____

Group	Fruits	Vegetables	Grains	Meat & Beans	Milk	Oils
Goal Amount						
Estimate Your Total						
Increase ⇧ or Decrease? ⇩						

Physical Activity: _____   Spiritual Activity: _____

Steps/Miles/Minutes: _____   _____

Day/Date: _____

Breakfast: _____   Lunch: _____

Dinner: _____   Snack: _____

Group	Fruits	Vegetables	Grains	Meat & Beans	Milk	Oils
Goal Amount						
Estimate Your Total						
Increase ⇧ or Decrease? ⇩						

Physical Activity: _____   Spiritual Activity: _____

Steps/Miles/Minutes: _____   _____

Day/Date: _____

Breakfast: _____   Lunch: _____

Dinner: _____   Snack: _____

Group	Fruits	Vegetables	Grains	Meat & Beans	Milk	Oils
Goal Amount						
Estimate Your Total						
Increase ⇧ or Decrease? ⇩						

Physical Activity: _____   Spiritual Activity: _____

Steps/Miles/Minutes: _____   _____

Day/Date:

Breakfast: _____ Lunch: _____

Dinner: _____ Snack: _____

Group	Fruits	Vegetables	Grains	Meat & Beans	Milk	Oils
Goal Amount						
Estimate Your Total						
Increase ⇧ or Decrease? ⇩						

Physical Activity: _____ Spiritual Activity: _____

Steps/Miles/Minutes: _____ _____

Day/Date:

Breakfast: _____ Lunch: _____

Dinner: _____ Snack: _____

Group	Fruits	Vegetables	Grains	Meat & Beans	Milk	Oils
Goal Amount						
Estimate Your Total						
Increase ⇧ or Decrease? ⇩						

Physical Activity: _____ Spiritual Activity: _____

Steps/Miles/Minutes: _____ _____

Day/Date:

Breakfast: _____ Lunch: _____

Dinner: _____ Snack: _____

Group	Fruits	Vegetables	Grains	Meat & Beans	Milk	Oils
Goal Amount						
Estimate Your Total						
Increase ⇧ or Decrease? ⇩						

Physical Activity: _____ Spiritual Activity: _____

Steps/Miles/Minutes: _____ _____

Day/Date:

Breakfast: _____ Lunch: _____

Dinner: _____ Snack: _____

Group	Fruits	Vegetables	Grains	Meat & Beans	Milk	Oils
Goal Amount						
Estimate Your Total						
Increase ⇧ or Decrease? ⇩						

Physical Activity: _____ Spiritual Activity: _____

Steps/Miles/Minutes: _____ _____

Live It Tracker

Name: _____ Loss/gain: _____ lbs.

Date: _____ Week #: _____ Calorie Range: _____ My food goal for next week: _____

Activity Level: None, < 30 min/day, 30-60 min/day, 60+ min/day My activity goal for next week: _____

Group	Daily Calories							
	1300-1400	1500-1600	1700-1800	1900-2000	2100-2200	2300-2400	2500-2600	2700-2800
Fruits	1.5-2 c.	1.5-2 c.	1.5-2 c.	2-2.5 c.	2-2.5 c.	2.5-3.5 c.	3.5-4.5 c.	3.5-4.5 c.
Vegetables	1.5-2 c.	2-2.5 c.	2.5-3 c.	2.5-3 c.	3-3.5 c.	3.5-4.5 c.	4.5-5 c.	4.5-5 c.
Grains	5 oz-eq.	5-6 oz-eq.	6-7 oz-eq.	6-7 oz-eq.	7-8 oz-eq.	8-9 oz-eq.	9-10 oz-eq.	10-11 oz-eq.
Meat & Beans	4 oz-eq.	5 oz-eq.	5-5.5 oz-eq.	5.5-6.5 oz-eq.	6.5-7 oz-eq.	7-7.5 oz-eq.	7-7.5 oz-eq.	7.5-8 oz-eq.
Milk	2-3 c.	3 c.	3 c.	3 c.	3 c.	3 c.	3 c.	3 c.
Healthy Oils	4 tsp.	5 tsp.	5 tsp.	6 tsp.	6 tsp.	7 tsp.	8 tsp.	8 tsp.

Day/Date:

Breakfast: _____ Lunch: _____

Dinner: _____ Snack: _____

Group	Fruits	Vegetables	Grains	Meat & Beans	Milk	Oils
Goal Amount						
Estimate Your Total						
Increase ⬆ or Decrease? ⬇						

Physical Activity: _____ Spiritual Activity: _____

Steps/Miles/Minutes: _____

Day/Date:

Breakfast: _____ Lunch: _____

Dinner: _____ Snack: _____

Group	Fruits	Vegetables	Grains	Meat & Beans	Milk	Oils
Goal Amount						
Estimate Your Total						
Increase ⬆ or Decrease? ⬇						

Physical Activity: _____ Spiritual Activity: _____

Steps/Miles/Minutes: _____

Day/Date:

Breakfast: _____ Lunch: _____

Dinner: _____ Snack: _____

Group	Fruits	Vegetables	Grains	Meat & Beans	Milk	Oils
Goal Amount						
Estimate Your Total						
Increase ⬆ or Decrease? ⬇						

Physical Activity: _____ Spiritual Activity: _____

Steps/Miles/Minutes: _____

Day/Date: _____

Breakfast: _____ Lunch: _____

Dinner: _____ Snack: _____

_____ _____

Group	Fruits	Vegetables	Grains	Meat & Beans	Milk	Oils
Goal Amount						
Estimate Your Total						
Increase ⇧ or Decrease? ⇩						

Physical Activity: _____ Spiritual Activity: _____

Steps/Miles/Minutes: _____ _____

Day/Date: _____

Breakfast: _____ Lunch: _____

Dinner: _____ Snack: _____

_____ _____

Group	Fruits	Vegetables	Grains	Meat & Beans	Milk	Oils
Goal Amount						
Estimate Your Total						
Increase ⇧ or Decrease? ⇩						

Physical Activity: _____ Spiritual Activity: _____

Steps/Miles/Minutes: _____ _____

Day/Date: _____

Breakfast: _____ Lunch: _____

Dinner: _____ Snack: _____

_____ _____

Group	Fruits	Vegetables	Grains	Meat & Beans	Milk	Oils
Goal Amount						
Estimate Your Total						
Increase ⇧ or Decrease? ⇩						

Physical Activity: _____ Spiritual Activity: _____

Steps/Miles/Minutes: _____ _____

Day/Date: _____

Breakfast: _____ Lunch: _____

Dinner: _____ Snack: _____

_____ _____

Group	Fruits	Vegetables	Grains	Meat & Beans	Milk	Oils
Goal Amount						
Estimate Your Total						
Increase ⇧ or Decrease? ⇩						

Physical Activity: _____ Spiritual Activity: _____

Steps/Miles/Minutes: _____ _____

Live It Tracker

Name: _____ Loss/gain: _____ lbs.

Date: _____ Week #: _____ Calorie Range: _____ My food goal for next week: _____

Activity Level: None, < 30 min/day, 30-60 min/day, 60+ min/day My activity goal for next week: _____

Group	Daily Calories							
	1300-1400	1500-1600	1700-1800	1900-2000	2100-2200	2300-2400	2500-2600	2700-2800
Fruits	1.5-2 c.	1.5-2 c.	1.5-2 c.	2-2.5 c.	2-2.5 c.	2.5-3.5 c.	3.5-4.5 c.	3.5-4.5 c.
Vegetables	1.5-2 c.	2-2.5 c.	2.5-3 c.	2.5-3 c.	3-3.5 c.	3.5-4.5 c.	4.5-5 c.	4.5-5 c.
Grains	5 oz-eq.	5-6 oz-eq.	6-7 oz-eq.	6-7 oz-eq.	7-8 oz-eq.	8-9 oz-eq.	9-10 oz-eq.	10-11 oz-eq.
Meat & Beans	4 oz-eq.	5 oz-eq.	5-5.5 oz-eq.	5.5-6.5 oz-eq.	6.5-7 oz-eq.	7-7.5 oz-eq.	7-7.5 oz-eq.	7.5-8 oz-eq.
Milk	2-3 c.	3 c.	3 c.	3 c.	3 c.	3 c.	3 c.	3 c.
Healthy Oils	4 tsp.	5 tsp.	5 tsp.	6 tsp.	6 tsp.	7 tsp.	8 tsp.	8 tsp.

Breakfast: _____   Lunch: _____

Dinner: _____   Snack: _____

Day/Date: _____

Group	Fruits	Vegetables	Grains	Meat & Beans	Milk	Oils
Goal Amount						
Estimate Your Total						
Increase ⇧ or Decrease? ⇩						

Physical Activity: _____   Spiritual Activity: _____

Steps/Miles/Minutes: _____

Breakfast: _____   Lunch: _____

Dinner: _____   Snack: _____

Day/Date: _____

Group	Fruits	Vegetables	Grains	Meat & Beans	Milk	Oils
Goal Amount						
Estimate Your Total						
Increase ⇧ or Decrease? ⇩						

Physical Activity: _____   Spiritual Activity: _____

Steps/Miles/Minutes: _____

Breakfast: _____   Lunch: _____

Dinner: _____   Snack: _____

Day/Date: _____

Group	Fruits	Vegetables	Grains	Meat & Beans	Milk	Oils
Goal Amount						
Estimate Your Total						
Increase ⇧ or Decrease? ⇩						

Physical Activity: _____   Spiritual Activity: _____

Steps/Miles/Minutes: _____

Day/Date: _____

Breakfast: _____ Lunch: _____

Dinner: _____ Snack: _____

Group	Fruits	Vegetables	Grains	Meat & Beans	Milk	Oils
Goal Amount						
Estimate Your Total						
Increase ⇧ or Decrease? ⇩						

Physical Activity: _____ Spiritual Activity: _____

Steps/Miles/Minutes: _____

Day/Date: _____

Breakfast: _____ Lunch: _____

Dinner: _____ Snack: _____

Group	Fruits	Vegetables	Grains	Meat & Beans	Milk	Oils
Goal Amount						
Estimate Your Total						
Increase ⇧ or Decrease? ⇩						

Physical Activity: _____ Spiritual Activity: _____

Steps/Miles/Minutes: _____

Day/Date: _____

Breakfast: _____ Lunch: _____

Dinner: _____ Snack: _____

Group	Fruits	Vegetables	Grains	Meat & Beans	Milk	Oils
Goal Amount						
Estimate Your Total						
Increase ⇧ or Decrease? ⇩						

Physical Activity: _____ Spiritual Activity: _____

Steps/Miles/Minutes: _____

Day/Date: _____

Breakfast: _____ Lunch: _____

Dinner: _____ Snack: _____

Group	Fruits	Vegetables	Grains	Meat & Beans	Milk	Oils
Goal Amount						
Estimate Your Total						
Increase ⇧ or Decrease? ⇩						

Physical Activity: _____ Spiritual Activity: _____

Steps/Miles/Minutes: _____

Live It Tracker

Name: _____ Loss/gain: _____ lbs.

Date: _____ Week #: ____ Calorie Range: _____ My food goal for next week: _____

Activity Level: None, < 30 min/day, 30-60 min/day, 60+ min/day My activity goal for next week: _____

Group	Daily Calories							
	1300-1400	1500-1600	1700-1800	1900-2000	2100-2200	2300-2400	2500-2600	2700-2800
Fruits	1.5-2 c.	1.5-2 c.	1.5-2 c.	2-2.5 c.	2-2.5 c.	2.5-3.5 c.	3.5-4.5 c.	3.5-4.5 c.
Vegetables	1.5-2 c.	2-2.5 c.	2.5-3 c.	2.5-3 c.	3-3.5 c.	3.5-4.5 c.	4.5-5 c.	4.5-5 c.
Grains	5 oz-eq.	5-6 oz-eq.	6-7 oz-eq.	6-7 oz-eq.	7-8 oz-eq.	8-9 oz-eq.	9-10 oz-eq.	10-11 oz-eq.
Meat & Beans	4 oz-eq.	5 oz-eq.	5-5.5 oz-eq.	5.5-6.5 oz-eq.	6.5-7 oz-eq.	7-7.5 oz-eq.	7-7.5 oz-eq.	7.5-8 oz-eq.
Milk	2-3 c.	3 c.	3 c.	3 c.	3 c.	3 c.	3 c.	3 c.
Healthy Oils	4 tsp.	5 tsp.	5 tsp.	6 tsp.	6 tsp.	7 tsp.	8 tsp.	8 tsp.

Day/Date:

Breakfast: _____ Lunch: _____

Dinner: _____ Snack: _____

Group	Fruits	Vegetables	Grains	Meat & Beans	Milk	Oils
Goal Amount						
Estimate Your Total						
Increase ⇧ or Decrease? ⇩						

Physical Activity: _____ Spiritual Activity: _____

Steps/Miles/Minutes: _____

Day/Date:

Breakfast: _____ Lunch: _____

Dinner: _____ Snack: _____

Group	Fruits	Vegetables	Grains	Meat & Beans	Milk	Oils
Goal Amount						
Estimate Your Total						
Increase ⇧ or Decrease? ⇩						

Physical Activity: _____ Spiritual Activity: _____

Steps/Miles/Minutes: _____

Day/Date:

Breakfast: _____ Lunch: _____

Dinner: _____ Snack: _____

Group	Fruits	Vegetables	Grains	Meat & Beans	Milk	Oils
Goal Amount						
Estimate Your Total						
Increase ⇧ or Decrease? ⇩						

Physical Activity: _____ Spiritual Activity: _____

Steps/Miles/Minutes: _____

Day/Date:

Breakfast: _____   Lunch: _____

Dinner: _____   Snack: _____

Group	Fruits	Vegetables	Grains	Meat & Beans	Milk	Oils
Goal Amount						
Estimate Your Total						
Increase ⬆ or Decrease? ⬇						

Physical Activity: _____   Spiritual Activity: _____

Steps/Miles/Minutes: _____

Day/Date:

Breakfast: _____   Lunch: _____

Dinner: _____   Snack: _____

Group	Fruits	Vegetables	Grains	Meat & Beans	Milk	Oils
Goal Amount						
Estimate Your Total						
Increase ⬆ or Decrease? ⬇						

Physical Activity: _____   Spiritual Activity: _____

Steps/Miles/Minutes: _____

Day/Date:

Breakfast: _____   Lunch: _____

Dinner: _____   Snack: _____

Group	Fruits	Vegetables	Grains	Meat & Beans	Milk	Oils
Goal Amount						
Estimate Your Total						
Increase ⬆ or Decrease? ⬇						

Physical Activity: _____   Spiritual Activity: _____

Steps/Miles/Minutes: _____

Day/Date:

Breakfast: _____   Lunch: _____

Dinner: _____   Snack: _____

Group	Fruits	Vegetables	Grains	Meat & Beans	Milk	Oils
Goal Amount						
Estimate Your Total						
Increase ⬆ or Decrease? ⬇						

Physical Activity: _____   Spiritual Activity: _____

Steps/Miles/Minutes: _____

Live It Tracker

Name: _____ Loss/gain: _____ lbs.

Date: _____ Week #: ____ Calorie Range: _____ My food goal for next week: _____

Activity Level: None, < 30 min/day, 30-60 min/day, 60+ min/day My activity goal for next week: _____

Group	Daily Calories							
	1300-1400	1500-1600	1700-1800	1900-2000	2100-2200	2300-2400	2500-2600	2700-2800
Fruits	1.5-2 c.	1.5-2 c.	1.5-2 c.	2-2.5 c.	2-2.5 c.	2.5-3.5 c.	3.5-4.5 c.	3.5-4.5 c.
Vegetables	1.5-2 c.	2-2.5 c.	2.5-3 c.	2.5-3 c.	3-3.5 c.	3.5-4.5 c.	4.5-5 c.	4.5-5 c.
Grains	5 oz-eq.	5-6 oz-eq.	6-7 oz-eq.	6-7 oz-eq.	7-8 oz-eq.	8-9 oz-eq.	9-10 oz-eq.	10-11 oz-eq.
Meat & Beans	4 oz-eq.	5 oz-eq.	5-5.5 oz-eq.	5.5-6.5 oz-eq.	6.5-7 oz-eq.	7-7.5 oz-eq.	7-7.5 oz-eq.	7.5-8 oz-eq.
Milk	2-3 c.	3 c.	3 c.	3 c.	3 c.	3 c.	3 c.	3 c.
Healthy Oils	4 tsp.	5 tsp.	5 tsp.	6 tsp.	6 tsp.	7 tsp.	8 tsp.	8 tsp.

Day/Date: _____

Breakfast: _____ Lunch: _____

Dinner: _____ Snack: _____

Group	Fruits	Vegetables	Grains	Meat & Beans	Milk	Oils
Goal Amount						
Estimate Your Total						
Increase ⇧ or Decrease? ⇩						

Physical Activity: _____ Spiritual Activity: _____

Steps/Miles/Minutes: _____

Day/Date: _____

Breakfast: _____ Lunch: _____

Dinner: _____ Snack: _____

Group	Fruits	Vegetables	Grains	Meat & Beans	Milk	Oils
Goal Amount						
Estimate Your Total						
Increase ⇧ or Decrease? ⇩						

Physical Activity: _____ Spiritual Activity: _____

Steps/Miles/Minutes: _____

Day/Date: _____

Breakfast: _____ Lunch: _____

Dinner: _____ Snack: _____

Group	Fruits	Vegetables	Grains	Meat & Beans	Milk	Oils
Goal Amount						
Estimate Your Total						
Increase ⇧ or Decrease? ⇩						

Physical Activity: _____ Spiritual Activity: _____

Steps/Miles/Minutes: _____

Breakfast: _____ **Lunch:** _____

Dinner: _____ **Snack:** _____

Group	Fruits	Vegetables	Grains	Meat & Beans	Milk	Oils
Goal Amount						
Estimate Your Total						
Increase ⬆ or Decrease? ⬇						

Physical Activity: _____ **Spiritual Activity:** _____

Steps/Miles/Minutes: _____ _____

Breakfast: _____ **Lunch:** _____

Dinner: _____ **Snack:** _____

Group	Fruits	Vegetables	Grains	Meat & Beans	Milk	Oils
Goal Amount						
Estimate Your Total						
Increase ⬆ or Decrease? ⬇						

Physical Activity: _____ **Spiritual Activity:** _____

Steps/Miles/Minutes: _____ _____

Breakfast: _____ **Lunch:** _____

Dinner: _____ **Snack:** _____

Group	Fruits	Vegetables	Grains	Meat & Beans	Milk	Oils
Goal Amount						
Estimate Your Total						
Increase ⬆ or Decrease? ⬇						

Physical Activity: _____ **Spiritual Activity:** _____

Steps/Miles/Minutes: _____ _____

Breakfast: _____ **Lunch:** _____

Dinner: _____ **Snack:** _____

Group	Fruits	Vegetables	Grains	Meat & Beans	Milk	Oils
Goal Amount						
Estimate Your Total						
Increase ⬆ or Decrease? ⬇						

Physical Activity: _____ **Spiritual Activity:** _____

Steps/Miles/Minutes: _____ _____

Day/Date:

Live It Tracker

Name: _____ Loss/gain: _____ lbs.

Date: _____ Week #: _____ Calorie Range: _____ My food goal for next week: _____

Activity Level: None, < 30 min/day, 30-60 min/day, 60+ min/day My activity goal for next week: _____

Group	Daily Calories							
	1300-1400	1500-1600	1700-1800	1900-2000	2100-2200	2300-2400	2500-2600	2700-2800
Fruits	1.5-2 c.	1.5-2 c.	1.5-2 c.	2-2.5 c.	2-2.5 c.	2.5-3.5 c.	3.5-4.5 c.	3.5-4.5 c.
Vegetables	1.5-2 c.	2-2.5 c.	2.5-3 c.	2.5-3 c.	3-3.5 c.	3.5-4.5 c.	4.5-5 c.	4.5-5 c.
Grains	5 oz-eq.	5-6 oz-eq.	6-7 oz-eq.	6-7 oz-eq.	7-8 oz-eq.	8-9 oz-eq.	9-10 oz-eq.	10-11 oz-eq.
Meat & Beans	4 oz-eq.	5 oz-eq.	5-5.5 oz-eq.	5.5-6.5 oz-eq.	6.5-7 oz-eq.	7-7.5 oz-eq.	7-7.5 oz-eq.	7.5-8 oz-eq.
Milk	2-3 c.	3 c.	3 c.	3 c.	3 c.	3 c.	3 c.	3 c.
Healthy Oils	4 tsp.	5 tsp.	5 tsp.	6 tsp.	6 tsp.	7 tsp.	8 tsp.	8 tsp.

Day/Date: _____

Breakfast: _____ Lunch: _____

Dinner: _____ Snack: _____

Group	Fruits	Vegetables	Grains	Meat & Beans	Milk	Oils
Goal Amount						
Estimate Your Total						
Increase ⇧ or Decrease? ⇩						

Physical Activity: _____ Spiritual Activity: _____

Steps/Miles/Minutes: _____

Day/Date: _____

Breakfast: _____ Lunch: _____

Dinner: _____ Snack: _____

Group	Fruits	Vegetables	Grains	Meat & Beans	Milk	Oils
Goal Amount						
Estimate Your Total						
Increase ⇧ or Decrease? ⇩						

Physical Activity: _____ Spiritual Activity: _____

Steps/Miles/Minutes: _____

Day/Date: _____

Breakfast: _____ Lunch: _____

Dinner: _____ Snack: _____

Group	Fruits	Vegetables	Grains	Meat & Beans	Milk	Oils
Goal Amount						
Estimate Your Total						
Increase ⇧ or Decrease? ⇩						

Physical Activity: _____ Spiritual Activity: _____

Steps/Miles/Minutes: _____

Day/Date: _____

Breakfast: _____	Lunch: _____
Dinner: _____	Snack: _____

Group	Fruits	Vegetables	Grains	Meat & Beans	Milk	Oils
Goal Amount						
Estimate Your Total						
Increase ⇧ or Decrease? ⇩						

Physical Activity: _____ Spiritual Activity: _____

Steps/Miles/Minutes: _____ _____

Day/Date: _____

Breakfast: _____	Lunch: _____
Dinner: _____	Snack: _____

Group	Fruits	Vegetables	Grains	Meat & Beans	Milk	Oils
Goal Amount						
Estimate Your Total						
Increase ⇧ or Decrease? ⇩						

Physical Activity: _____ Spiritual Activity: _____

Steps/Miles/Minutes: _____ _____

Day/Date: _____

Breakfast: _____	Lunch: _____
Dinner: _____	Snack: _____

Group	Fruits	Vegetables	Grains	Meat & Beans	Milk	Oils
Goal Amount						
Estimate Your Total						
Increase ⇧ or Decrease? ⇩						

Physical Activity: _____ Spiritual Activity: _____

Steps/Miles/Minutes: _____ _____

Day/Date: _____

Breakfast: _____	Lunch: _____
Dinner: _____	Snack: _____

Group	Fruits	Vegetables	Grains	Meat & Beans	Milk	Oils
Goal Amount						
Estimate Your Total						
Increase ⇧ or Decrease? ⇩						

Physical Activity: _____ Spiritual Activity: _____

Steps/Miles/Minutes: _____ _____

Live It Tracker

Name: _____ Loss/gain: _____ lbs.

Date: _____ Week #: _____ Calorie Range: _____ My food goal for next week: _____

Activity Level: None, < 30 min/day, 30-60 min/day, 60+ min/day My activity goal for next week: _____

Group	Daily Calories							
	1300-1400	1500-1600	1700-1800	1900-2000	2100-2200	2300-2400	2500-2600	2700-2800
Fruits	1.5-2 c.	1.5-2 c.	1.5-2 c.	2-2.5 c.	2-2.5 c.	2.5-3.5 c.	3.5-4.5 c.	3.5-4.5 c.
Vegetables	1.5-2 c.	2-2.5 c.	2.5-3 c.	2.5-3 c.	3-3.5 c.	3.5-4.5 c.	4.5-5 c.	4.5-5 c.
Grains	5 oz-eq.	5-6 oz-eq.	6-7 oz-eq.	6-7 oz-eq.	7-8 oz-eq.	8-9 oz-eq.	9-10 oz-eq.	10-11 oz-eq.
Meat & Beans	4 oz-eq.	5 oz-eq.	5-5.5 oz-eq.	5.5-6.5 oz-eq.	6.5-7 oz-eq.	7-7.5 oz-eq.	7-7.5 oz-eq.	7.5-8 oz-eq.
Milk	2-3 c.	3 c.	3 c.	3 c.	3 c.	3 c.	3 c.	3 c.
Healthy Oils	4 tsp.	5 tsp.	5 tsp.	6 tsp.	6 tsp.	7 tsp.	8 tsp.	8 tsp.

Day/Date: _____

Breakfast: _____ Lunch: _____

Dinner: _____ Snack: _____

Group	Fruits	Vegetables	Grains	Meat & Beans	Milk	Oils
Goal Amount						
Estimate Your Total						
Increase ⇧ or Decrease? ⇩						

Physical Activity: _____ Spiritual Activity: _____

Steps/Miles/Minutes: _____

Day/Date: _____

Breakfast: _____ Lunch: _____

Dinner: _____ Snack: _____

Group	Fruits	Vegetables	Grains	Meat & Beans	Milk	Oils
Goal Amount						
Estimate Your Total						
Increase ⇧ or Decrease? ⇩						

Physical Activity: _____ Spiritual Activity: _____

Steps/Miles/Minutes: _____

Day/Date: _____

Breakfast: _____ Lunch: _____

Dinner: _____ Snack: _____

Group	Fruits	Vegetables	Grains	Meat & Beans	Milk	Oils
Goal Amount						
Estimate Your Total						
Increase ⇧ or Decrease? ⇩						

Physical Activity: _____ Spiritual Activity: _____

Steps/Miles/Minutes: _____

Day/Date: _____

Breakfast: _____ Lunch: _____

Dinner: _____ Snack: _____

Group	Fruits	Vegetables	Grains	Meat & Beans	Milk	Oils
Goal Amount						
Estimate Your Total						
Increase ⇧ or Decrease? ⇩						

Physical Activity: _____ Spiritual Activity: _____

Steps/Miles/Minutes: _____ _____

Day/Date: _____

Breakfast: _____ Lunch: _____

Dinner: _____ Snack: _____

Group	Fruits	Vegetables	Grains	Meat & Beans	Milk	Oils
Goal Amount						
Estimate Your Total						
Increase ⇧ or Decrease? ⇩						

Physical Activity: _____ Spiritual Activity: _____

Steps/Miles/Minutes: _____ _____

Day/Date: _____

Breakfast: _____ Lunch: _____

Dinner: _____ Snack: _____

Group	Fruits	Vegetables	Grains	Meat & Beans	Milk	Oils
Goal Amount						
Estimate Your Total						
Increase ⇧ or Decrease? ⇩						

Physical Activity: _____ Spiritual Activity: _____

Steps/Miles/Minutes: _____ _____

Day/Date: _____

Breakfast: _____ Lunch: _____

Dinner: _____ Snack: _____

Group	Fruits	Vegetables	Grains	Meat & Beans	Milk	Oils
Goal Amount						
Estimate Your Total						
Increase ⇧ or Decrease? ⇩						

Physical Activity: _____ Spiritual Activity: _____

Steps/Miles/Minutes: _____ _____

Live It Tracker

Name: _____ Loss/gain: _____ lbs.

Date: _____ Week #: _____ Calorie Range: _____ My food goal for next week: _____

Activity Level: None, < 30 min/day, 30-60 min/day, 60+ min/day My activity goal for next week: _____

Group	Daily Calories							
	1300-1400	1500-1600	1700-1800	1900-2000	2100-2200	2300-2400	2500-2600	2700-2800
Fruits	1.5-2 c.	1.5-2 c.	1.5-2 c.	2-2.5 c.	2-2.5 c.	2.5-3.5 c.	3.5-4.5 c.	3.5-4.5 c.
Vegetables	1.5-2 c.	2-2.5 c.	2.5-3 c.	2.5-3 c.	3-3.5 c.	3.5-4.5 c.	4.5-5 c.	4.5-5 c.
Grains	5 oz-eq.	5-6 oz-eq.	6-7 oz-eq.	6-7 oz-eq.	7-8 oz-eq.	8-9 oz-eq.	9-10 oz-eq.	10-11 oz-eq.
Meat & Beans	4 oz-eq.	5 oz-eq.	5-5.5 oz-eq.	5.5-6.5 oz-eq.	6.5-7 oz-eq.	7-7.5 oz-eq.	7-7.5 oz-eq.	7.5-8 oz-eq.
Milk	2-3 c.	3 c.	3 c.	3 c.	3 c.	3 c.	3 c.	3 c.
Healthy Oils	4 tsp.	5 tsp.	5 tsp.	6 tsp.	6 tsp.	7 tsp.	8 tsp.	8 tsp.

Day/Date:

Breakfast: _____ Lunch: _____

Dinner: _____ Snack: _____

Group	Fruits	Vegetables	Grains	Meat & Beans	Milk	Oils
Goal Amount						
Estimate Your Total						
Increase ⇧ or Decrease? ⇩						

Physical Activity: _____ Spiritual Activity: _____

Steps/Miles/Minutes: _____

Day/Date:

Breakfast: _____ Lunch: _____

Dinner: _____ Snack: _____

Group	Fruits	Vegetables	Grains	Meat & Beans	Milk	Oils
Goal Amount						
Estimate Your Total						
Increase ⇧ or Decrease? ⇩						

Physical Activity: _____ Spiritual Activity: _____

Steps/Miles/Minutes: _____

Day/Date:

Breakfast: _____ Lunch: _____

Dinner: _____ Snack: _____

Group	Fruits	Vegetables	Grains	Meat & Beans	Milk	Oils
Goal Amount						
Estimate Your Total						
Increase ⇧ or Decrease? ⇩						

Physical Activity: _____ Spiritual Activity: _____

Steps/Miles/Minutes: _____

Day/Date: ___

Breakfast: _____ Lunch: _____

Dinner: _____ Snack: _____

Group	Fruits	Vegetables	Grains	Meat & Beans	Milk	Oils
Goal Amount						
Estimate Your Total						
Increase ⬆ or Decrease? ⬇						

Physical Activity: _____ Spiritual Activity: _____

Steps/Miles/Minutes: _____ _____

Day/Date: ___

Breakfast: _____ Lunch: _____

Dinner: _____ Snack: _____

Group	Fruits	Vegetables	Grains	Meat & Beans	Milk	Oils
Goal Amount						
Estimate Your Total						
Increase ⬆ or Decrease? ⬇						

Physical Activity: _____ Spiritual Activity: _____

Steps/Miles/Minutes: _____ _____

Day/Date: ___

Breakfast: _____ Lunch: _____

Dinner: _____ Snack: _____

Group	Fruits	Vegetables	Grains	Meat & Beans	Milk	Oils
Goal Amount						
Estimate Your Total						
Increase ⬆ or Decrease? ⬇						

Physical Activity: _____ Spiritual Activity: _____

Steps/Miles/Minutes: _____ _____

Day/Date: ___

Breakfast: _____ Lunch: _____

Dinner: _____ Snack: _____

Group	Fruits	Vegetables	Grains	Meat & Beans	Milk	Oils
Goal Amount						
Estimate Your Total						
Increase ⬆ or Decrease? ⬇						

Physical Activity: _____ Spiritual Activity: _____

Steps/Miles/Minutes: _____ _____

Live It Tracker

Name: _____ Loss/gain: _____ lbs.

Date: _____ Week #: _____ Calorie Range: _____ My food goal for next week: _____

Activity Level: None, < 30 min/day, 30-60 min/day, 60+ min/day My activity goal for next week: _____

Group	Daily Calories							
	1300-1400	1500-1600	1700-1800	1900-2000	2100-2200	2300-2400	2500-2600	2700-2800
Fruits	1.5-2 c.	1.5-2 c.	1.5-2 c.	2-2.5 c.	2-2.5 c.	2.5-3.5 c.	3.5-4.5 c.	3.5-4.5 c.
Vegetables	1.5-2 c.	2-2.5 c.	2.5-3 c.	2.5-3 c.	3-3.5 c.	3.5-4.5 c.	4.5-5 c.	4.5-5 c.
Grains	5 oz-eq.	5-6 oz-eq.	6-7 oz-eq.	6-7 oz-eq.	7-8 oz-eq.	8-9 oz-eq.	9-10 oz-eq.	10-11 oz-eq.
Meat & Beans	4 oz-eq.	5 oz-eq.	5-5.5 oz-eq.	5.5-6.5 oz-eq.	6.5-7 oz-eq.	7-7.5 oz-eq.	7-7.5 oz-eq.	7.5-8 oz-eq.
Milk	2-3 c.	3 c.	3 c.	3 c.	3 c.	3 c.	3 c.	3 c.
Healthy Oils	4 tsp.	5 tsp.	5 tsp.	6 tsp.	6 tsp.	7 tsp.	8 tsp.	8 tsp.

Day/Date:

Breakfast: _____ Lunch: _____

Dinner: _____ Snack: _____

Group	Fruits	Vegetables	Grains	Meat & Beans	Milk	Oils
Goal Amount						
Estimate Your Total						
Increase ⇧ or Decrease? ⇩						

Physical Activity: _____ Spiritual Activity: _____

Steps/Miles/Minutes: _____

Day/Date:

Breakfast: _____ Lunch: _____

Dinner: _____ Snack: _____

Group	Fruits	Vegetables	Grains	Meat & Beans	Milk	Oils
Goal Amount						
Estimate Your Total						
Increase ⇧ or Decrease? ⇩						

Physical Activity: _____ Spiritual Activity: _____

Steps/Miles/Minutes: _____

Day/Date:

Breakfast: _____ Lunch: _____

Dinner: _____ Snack: _____

Group	Fruits	Vegetables	Grains	Meat & Beans	Milk	Oils
Goal Amount						
Estimate Your Total						
Increase ⇧ or Decrease? ⇩						

Physical Activity: _____ Spiritual Activity: _____

Steps/Miles/Minutes: _____

Day/Date:

Breakfast: _____ Lunch: _____

Dinner: _____ Snack: _____

Group	Fruits	Vegetables	Grains	Meat & Beans	Milk	Oils
Goal Amount						
Estimate Your Total						
Increase ⬆ or Decrease? ⬇						

Physical Activity: _____ Spiritual Activity: _____

Steps/Miles/Minutes: _____ _____

Day/Date:

Breakfast: _____ Lunch: _____

Dinner: _____ Snack: _____

Group	Fruits	Vegetables	Grains	Meat & Beans	Milk	Oils
Goal Amount						
Estimate Your Total						
Increase ⬆ or Decrease? ⬇						

Physical Activity: _____ Spiritual Activity: _____

Steps/Miles/Minutes: _____ _____

Day/Date:

Breakfast: _____ Lunch: _____

Dinner: _____ Snack: _____

Group	Fruits	Vegetables	Grains	Meat & Beans	Milk	Oils
Goal Amount						
Estimate Your Total						
Increase ⬆ or Decrease? ⬇						

Physical Activity: _____ Spiritual Activity: _____

Steps/Miles/Minutes: _____ _____

Day/Date:

Breakfast: _____ Lunch: _____

Dinner: _____ Snack: _____

Group	Fruits	Vegetables	Grains	Meat & Beans	Milk	Oils
Goal Amount						
Estimate Your Total						
Increase ⬆ or Decrease? ⬇						

Physical Activity: _____ Spiritual Activity: _____

Steps/Miles/Minutes: _____ _____

let's count our miles!

Join the 100-Mile Club this Session

Can't walk that mile yet? Don't be discouraged! There are exercises you can do to strengthen your body and burn those extra calories. Keep a record on your Live It Tracker of the number of minutes you do these common physical activities, convert those minutes to miles following the chart below, and then mark off each mile you have completed on the chart found on the back of the front cover. Report your miles to your 100-Mile Club representative when you first arrive each week. Remember, you are not competing with anyone else . . . just yourself. Your job is to strive to reach 100 miles before the last meeting in this session. You can do it—just keep on moving!

Walking

slowly, 2 mph	30 min. = 156 cal. = 1 mile
moderately, 3 mph	20 min. = 156 cal. = 1 mile
very briskly, 4 mph	15 min. = 156 cal. = 1 mile
speed walking	10 min. = 156 cal. = 1 mile
up stairs	13 min. = 159 cal. = 1 mile

Running/Jogging
10 min. = 156 cal. = 1 mile

Cycling Outdoors

slowly, <10 mph	20 min. = 156 cal. = 1 mile
light effort, 10-12 mph	12 min. = 156 cal. = 1 mile
moderate effort, 12-14 mph.	10 min. = 156 cal. = 1 mile
vigorous effort, 14-16 mph	7.5 min. = 156 cal. = 1 mile
very fast, 16-19 mph	6.5 min. = 152 cal. = 1 mile

Sports Activities

Playing tennis (singles)	10 min. = 156 cal. = 1 mile
Swimming	
light to moderate effort	11 min. = 152 cal. = 1 mile
fast, vigorous effort	7.5 min. = 156 cal. = 1 mile
Softball	15 min. = 156 cal. = 1 mile
Golf	20 min. = 156 cal = 1 mile
Rollerblading	6.5 min. = 152 cal. = 1 mile
Ice skating	11 min. = 152 cal. = 1 mile

Jumping rope	7.5 min. = 156 cal. = 1 mile
Basketball	12 min. = 156 cal. = 1 mile
Soccer (casual)	15 min. = 159 cal. = 1 mile

Around the House
Mowing grass	22 min. = 156 cal. = 1 mile
Mopping, sweeping, vacuuming	19.5 min. = 155 cal. = 1 mile
Cooking	40 min. =160 cal. = 1 mile
Gardening	19 min. = 156 cal. = 1 mile
Housework (general)	35 min. = 156 cal. = 1 mile
Ironing	45 min. = 153 cal. = 1 mile
Raking leaves	25 min. = 150 cal. = 1 mile
Washing car	23 min. = 156 cal. = 1 mile
Washing dishes	45 min. = 153 cal. = 1 mile

At the Gym
Stair machine	8.5 min. = 155 cal. = 1 mile
Stationary bike	
slowly, 10 mph	30 min. = 156 cal. = 1 mile
moderately, 10-13 mph	15 min. = 156 cal. = 1 mile
vigorously, 13-16 mph	7.5 min. = 156 cal. = 1 mile
briskly, 16-19 mph	6.5 min. = 156 cal. = 1 mile
Elliptical trainer	12 min. = 156 cal. = 1 mile
Weight machines (used vigorously)	13 min. = 152 cal.=1 mile
Aerobics	
low impact	15 min. = 156 cal. = 1 mile
high impact	12 min. = 156 cal. = 1 mile
water	20 min. = 156 cal. = 1 mile
Pilates	15 min. = 156 cal. = 1 mile
Raquetball (casual)	15 min. = 159 cal. = 1 mile
Stretching exercises	25 min. = 150 cal. = 1 mile
Weight lifting (also works for weight	
machines used moderately or gently)	30 min. = 156 cal. = 1 mile

Family Leisure
Playing piano	37 min. = 155 cal. = 1 mile
Jumping rope	10 min. = 152 cal. = 1 mile
Skating (moderate)	20 min. = 152 cal. = 1 mile
Swimming	
moderate	17 min. = 156 cal. = 1 mile
vigorous	10 min. = 148 cal. = 1 mile
Table tennis	25 min. = 150 cal. = 1 mile
Walk/run/play with kids	25 min. = 150 cal. = 1 mile